# THE MIND OF A MNEMONIST

*A Little Book*

*about a Vast Memory*

# THE MIND OF
# A MNEMONIST

## *A. R. Luria*

TRANSLATED FROM THE RUSSIAN
*by Lynn Solotaroff*

*With a new foreword by Jerome S. Bruner*

HARVARD UNIVERSITY PRESS
CAMBRIDGE, MASSACHUSETTS
AND LONDON, ENGLAND

LIBRARY OF CONGRESS CATALOGING-IN-PUBLICATION DATA
Luriia, A. R. (Aleksandr Romanovich), 1902–
    The mind of a mnemonist.

    Translation of: Malen'kaia knizhka o bol'shoĭ
pamiati.
    Reprint. Originally published: New York : Basic
Books, Inc., 1968. With new introd.
    Includes index.
    1. Memory, Disorders of — Case studies.
2. Memory.  I. Title.
BF376.L813   1987     616.85'8     86-31847
ISBN: 0-674-57622-5

... The time has come, the walrus said, to
talk of many things ...
LEWIS CARROLL
*Through the Looking-Glass*

... Together with little Alice we will slip
past the smooth, cold surface of the looking
glass and find ourselves in a wonderland,
where everything is at once so familiar and
recognizable, yet so strange and uncommon.

# CONTENTS

# FOREWORD
# TO THE
# 1987 EDITION

*Jerome S. Bruner*

Since its first publication some twenty years ago, this "little book," as Luria called it, has become a classic, a classic in two senses. It has, for one, become a classic in the clinical literature on pathologies of memory and on the significance of such pathologies for our understanding of memory in general. That, in its way, was not altogether unexpected, for Luria had already emerged in those years as one of the most gifted observers of the effects of neurological disorders on the workings of the human mind. He has since taken his place, as it were, in the ranks of the greats: Hughlings Jackson, Sir Henry Head, Kurt Goldstein, and that small band of clinical neurologists who have so deeply enriched our understanding of aphasias, amnesias, apraxias, and kindred afflictions. And today we can better understand the psychological acumen of

Luria's observations and insights, for our new knowledge of memory and its mechanisms have helped us recognize how much Luria in his time was a visitor from the future.

But there is a second sense, perhaps a more interesting sense, in which the book has become a classic. It can be said of it that it founded a genre, not so much a scientific genre, but a literary one. For it was not simply the technical penetration of Luria's observations that made the book a success, but the human quality, the compassion of the author in recognizing the human plight of his patient. This is not a cold, clinical account, but a humane interpretation of what it means for somebody to live with a mind that records meticulously the details of experience without being able, so to speak, to extract from the record what it means, "what it's all about." In this sense, Luria's humane yet naked account — he liked to call this genre "romantic science" — is in the spirit of a Kafka or a Beckett writing of characters who are symbolically dispossesed of the power to find meaning in the world. In his way, S., Luria's patient in this book, takes his place beside Joseph K. in *The Trial*, or in the gallery of lost souls that Beckett has brought to life in his stories and plays. In this new dispensation, "pathology" becomes not a domain alien to the human condition, but part of the human condition itself. Rather than dismissing the ill and the injured as beyond the pale of human explication, we ask instead about their subjective landscape, their implicit epistemology, their presuppositions. They cease being "cases" and become human beings again. And they become part of literature as well as science.

This new genre, this way of comprehending the consequences of man's bodily troubles not simply as "organic syndromes" but as human plights has, since the publication of Luria's classic books, attracted new and gifted voices. Oliver Sacks's *Awakenings* and the briefer case studies in his more recent *The Man Who Mistook His Wife for a Hat* were directly inspired by Luria. And Jonathan Miller has produced two moving and perceptive documentaries for the BBC, one on a severe Parkinsonian patient who is full of pluck and effort, the other on a Korsakoff patient clinging to his premorbid learnedness. Both films do not simply document "cases," but explicate human ordinariness and human courage in the face of crippling affliction. Even animal research on brain extirpation has been enriched, as in Nick Humphrey's classic study of the monkey "Helen," in which he explores not only her deficits, but also how her life was affected by them. In the tradition of Luria's studies, the investigator reaches out to the subject—more as a collaborator than as a test-wielding visitor to her cageside.

And so at last, impelled by Luria's spirit, we are learning to understand the deaf, the blind, the stroke victim, the amputee — to understand them as human beings coping or failing to cope with the human condition rather than simply having "a medical problem."

I rather suspect that the change, the invention of the new genre, also reflects a changing temper in philosophy, another chapter in the struggle to free the human sciences from the drab captivity of nineteenth-century Positivism. Explanation of any human condition is so bound to context, so complexly interpretive at so many levels, that it cannot be achieved by considering isolated segments of life in vitro, and it can never be, even at its best, brought to a final conclusion beyond the shadow of human doubt. For a human being is, indeed, not "an islande entire to himself." He lives in a web of transactions, and his powers and his tragedies grow out of his transactional life. Memory loss in old age, for example, has been shown to depend upon how demanding we are of the aged with respect to their memory. Similarly, a learned review by William Hirst indicates to what extent the restoration of memory in amnesia depends upon the will of the sufferer to find indirect routes into his disturbed memory store—which depends again on what the sufferer is like as a human being and how supported he feels in his efforts by the world around him.

I think Luria was among the first to see these matters clearly, and certainly among the first to have the courage to write in this temper. He speaks of these efforts—particularly in his two great case histories, *The Man with a Shattered World* and *The Mind of a Mnemonist*—as "romantic science." It is worth a moment's pause to try to understand why he uses such an odd expression, for he surely must have known that it was likely to be misunderstood.

Indeed, both the term and the works that Luria describes as falling into the "romantic" category have been not so much misunderstood as ignored in most standard "hard-nosed" commentaries on his work. The admirable Harvard edition of Luria's intellectual autobiography, *The Making of Mind*, does not list either book in its bibliography of his "major works in English," and Michael Cole in his sensitive epilogue to that volume, "A Portrait of Luria," passes over this aspect of his life work with virtually no comment. Yet, reading that final chapter of his autobiography, the one entitled "Romantic Science," leaves one with the conclusion that this was not simply one of his "topics," but one of Luria's central philosophical concerns from the start.

A few passages will serve to illustrate. In that final autobiographical chapter he contrasts "classical" and "romantic" science (or scientists). The first is dedicated to the analysis of "living reality" into its constituent elements, with the object of formulating "abstract general laws" to which elementary phenomena can be referred. "One outcome of this approach is the reduction of living reality with all its richness of detail to abstract schema," he explains. "Romantics in science want neither to split living reality into its elementary components nor to represent the wealth of life's concrete events in abstract models that lose the properties of the phenomena themselves." Discussing the hazards of an excessive enthusiasm for either of the two extremes, he notes: "I have long puzzled over which of the two approaches, in principle, leads to a better understanding of living reality" and confesses that the issue had "concerned me during the first years of my intellectual life." In fact, "one of the major factors that drew me to Vygotsky was his emphasis on the necessity to resolve this crisis."

He then points to the ravaging effects of abstract learning theory in psychology: "the rich and complex picture of human behavior which existed in the late nineteenth century disappeared from psychology textbooks." And when electronic recording devices made it possible to detect more and more elementary units that were not accessible to the unaided human observer, the enthusiasm for abstract analysis without regard for rich context grew almost out of hand. Finally, he says ruefully, computers were developed that could submit these electronic observations to swift and complex mathematical analysis. "Many scholars began to suppose that observation could be replaced by computer simulation and mathematical models. Psychological textbooks overflowed with such models and schemas. This deluge brought a still greater danger: the reality of human conscious activity was being replaced by mechanical models." And then the interpretivist in Luria speaks out: "Scientific observation is not merely pure description of separate facts. Its main goal is to view an event from as many perspectives as possible." In the end, we must find the "inner laws" that produce the uniqueness of each event in its setting; we must finally (in words he borrows from Karl Marx) "ascend to the concrete."

Of his two classic case histories, he remarks, "In each of these works I tried to follow in the steps of Walter Pater in *Imaginary Portraits*, written in 1887, except that my books were *unimagined* portraits. In both books I described an individual and the laws of his life." Indeed, "a description of Sherashevsky [the mnemonist] would have been inadequate if it had been limited to his memory. What was required was an analysis of how his fantastic memory influenced his thinking, his behavior, and his personality." And for this Luria needed the full thirty years of collaborative observation that he and Sherashevsky devoted to the case.

All of that is plain enough, and there is little doubt that "romantic science" was no foible of Luria's later years. But let one other thing be clear. "Romantic" Luria may have been — searching out the uniqueness of this afflicted man with his cripplingly prodigious memory and his image-dominated mode of coping. But there runs through this book (and through *The Man with a Shattered World* as well) two crucial conceptual ideas that characterize Luria as a "classical" scientist. Through all his work, experimental and clinical alike, Luria was convinced that the aim of mental functioning was to construct two complementary versions of the same world. Indeed, he urged that the human nervous system is structured in a manner to help us achieve this dual representation and to help us put the two representations together. One is a simultaneous world in which, as in a panorama, we catch "on the fly" what is needed of what is there. The other is a temporally organized world that is structured around plans and intentions, a world made possible by the frontal cortical system. Frontal lesions disrupt intentionality and planfulness; occipital and parieto-temporal ones produce such anomalies as "simultanagnosia," in which elements and features can be isolated, but a "whole" or meaningful picture cannot be put together. Like his teacher Vygotsky, Luria believed that language plays a crucial role in bringing the two spheres together.

In the pages that follow, the reader will see many variations on these two themes. In S.'s case, the rich synesthesia of his memory images, their very completeness, prevents his fusing the simultaneous with time-contextualized planning, as if one system won out over the other, or a hypertrophy of one prevented the other from developing.

I mention these matters only to make the point that Luria, the "romantic" narrativist, was not only on good terms with Luria the "classic" scientist, but the two of them were working hand in glove to resolve the crisis to which Vygotsky had awakened the young Luria. Yet I doubt he ever felt that he could reconcile the two, but he used each to elucidate the other—not just in his two great case histories but throughout his scientific life. For him, as for his great teacher, the reconciliation of the two ways of using mind remained the "great crisis" of psychology. And I think it was so for him in principle.

Perhaps I can best illustrate it with an anecdote. I recall walking with Luria on one of our last visits together a year or two before his death in 1977. It was in Brussels and we were discussing a Vygotskian dilemma. It was the issue of how inventions in language and culture led to an unfolding of unsuspected potentialities in man, since mind grew by the incorporation of cultural and historical innovation. "It is vanity," I recall him saying, "to dream of having a completely predictive psychology, given man and history as they are and as they might one day be. But perhaps it is the best we can do as we do now: to understand what we can and have inspired ideas that lead us to observe the rest with care." My own guess is that his "inspired ideas" and his brilliant observations grew out of his romantic science, not just in those last two books, but from the start. And that is probably why he begins the last chapter in his autobiography with the famous quotation from Goethe: "Gray is all theory; green grows the golden tree of life."

But that does not quite catch it all, and it certainly misses out on one ingredient that makes this book such a human document. There was a compassionate side to Luria, and it shines through the two case books. For Luria was not simply trying to understand these two men, the one with a grossly hypertrophied memory, the other with a penetrating bullet fragment in the left parieto-occipital area of his cranium. He was trying to bring them back to some fullness of life. And that is what nourished his zest for observation, that and an insatiable scientific curiosity. It is not amiss to remark here that Luria, more than any of his contemporaries, believed in and worked devotedly on the rehabilitation of the brain-injured. And he believed that he could help those two men, and while he was perhaps more successful with "the man with a shattered world" than he was with S., he helped them both. Niels Bohr once remarked, in a quite different context, how difficult it was to know somebody both in the light of love and in the light of justice — indeed, he argued the impossibility of reconciling them. Luria was a physician as well as a scientist, and one sometimes has reason to wonder whether those two ideals, like love and justice, might also be irreconcilable. But great man that he was, he pursued them both. And perhaps after all, as the French proverb has it, the road is better than the inn.

# FOREWORD
# TO THE
# FIRST EDITION

*Jerome S. Bruner*

This book is an extraordinary tribute to Aleksandr Romanovich Luria. The richness of clinical insight, the acuity of the observations, and the fullness of the over-all picture of his mnemonist are all extraordinary. Luria tells us that he is treating the "case" as a study of a syndrome, a type of study in which he is especially skilled, as we know from his fine work on various patterns of brain lesions. What emerges is a perceptive study not only of memory organization but also of the manner in which memory is imbedded in a pattern of life. As a contribution to the clinical literature on memory pathology, this book will surely rank as a classic.

Though the title of this book suggests a study of great feats of memory, it is in fact a book about the failure of one aspect of memory and the hypertrophy of another. For the mnemonist, S., whose case is studied in such exquisite detail in these pages, is a man whose memory is a memory of particulars, particulars that are rich in imagery, thematic elaboation, and affect. But it is a memory that is peculiarly lacking in one important feature: the capacity to convert encounters with the particular into instances of the general, enabling one to form general concepts even though the particulars are lost. It is this latter type of "memory without record" that seems so poorly developed in this man.

Several notable things about the disorders of this mnemonist are especially fascinating from a psychological point of view. For one thing, the sheer persistence of ikonic memory is so great that one wonders whether there is some failure in the swift metabolism of short-term memory. His "immediate" images haunt him for hours, types of images that in much recent work on short-term memory are found to fade to a point where information retrieval from them is not possible after a second or so. Along with this trait there is also a non-selectivity about his memory, such that what remains behind is a kind of junk heap of impressions. Or perhaps this mnemonic disarray results from the evident failure to organize and "regularize" what is remembered into the kinds of schemata that Bartlett described in such detail in his classic *Remembering*. Curiously enough, and typically, our mnemonist has great difficulty organizing disparate encounters in terms of invariant features that characterize them.

The gift of persistent, concrete memory appears to make for highly concrete thinking, a kind of thinking in images that is very reminiscent of young children whose thought processes my colleagues and I have been studying (e.g., in *Studies in Cognitive Growth*, 1966). S.'s grouping of objects and words are thematic, associative, bound in a flow of edge-related images, almost with a feeling of naïve poetry. "... *A zhuk*—that's a dented piece in the potty ... It's a piece of rye bread ... And in the evening when you turn on the light, that's also *a zhuk*, for the entire room isn't lit up, just a small area, while everything else remains dark, *a zhuk*. Warts are also *a zhuk* ... Now I see them sitting me before a mirror. There's noise, laughter. There are my eyes staring at me from the mirror—dark— they're also *a zhuk*." So the mnemonist tries to define a childhood phrase he recalls at one of his sessions. But though the account has a kind of naïve poetry, it is misleading to think of the gift of poetry as within this man's reach. In fact, he has great difficulty in understanding some poems of Pasternak that were used for testing. He cannot get behind the surface images; he seems to be caught with the superficial meanings of words and cannot deal with their intended metaphor.

So powerful is his imagery that this man can easily drive his pulse up by imagining running. He is flooded and disturbed by the images and impressions of childhood, and, when he was a child, his imagery of school would become so "real" that he would lie abed rather than get out from under the quilt and get ready. It is interesting that, given his mode of remembering, there seems to be no childhood amnesia, and his memories from the earliest period can cause him acute malaise and chagrin. Throughout, there is a childlike quality in the protocols, protocols that are rich beyond anything I have ever encountered in the psychological literature on memory disorders. S.'s life in some deeply touching way is a failure. He waited for something to happen to him, some great thing. In the conduct of his life, too, there was a passive-receptive attitude, almost precluding organized striving. In place of the more abstract and constructional attitude of planning, there was waiting.

In writing this foreword, I cannot forgo one personal remark. I am among those who have been fortunate enough to have examined patients with Professor Luria at the Budenko Neurological Hospital in Moscow. It is an experience never to be forgotten, for his subtle capacity for bringing important material to light by ingenious questions and novel procedures is truly remarkable. It was no less so in the 1920's, when this study began. What is evident in this early work, as in his most recent work, is Professor Luria's ability to combine the clinical wisdom of the fine physician with the theoretical acumen of the scientific psychologist. May these talents be more widely spread among us in the future. Perhaps this book will encourage others like it.

*Cambridge, Mass.*
*October 21, 1967*

# PREFACE

I spent this summer off in the country, away from the city. Through the open windows I could hear the leaves rustling on the trees and catch the fragrant smell of grass. On my desk lay some old, yellowed notes from which I put together this brief account of a strange individual: a Jewish boy who, having failed as a musician and as a journalist, had become a mnemonist, met with many prominent people, yet remained a somewhat anchorless person, living with the expectation that at any moment something particularly fine was to come his way. He taught me and my friends a great deal, and it is only right that this book be dedicated to his memory.

A. R. L.

*Summer 1965*

# THE MIND OF A MNEMONIST

# 1

## *Introduction*

This brief account of a man's vast memory has quite a history behind it. For almost thirty years the author had an opportunity systematically to observe a man whose remarkable memory was one of the keenest the literature on the subject has ever described.

During this time the enormous amount of material which was assembled made it possible not only to explore the main patterns and devices of the man's memory (which for all practical purposes was inexhaustible), but to delineate the distinct personality features this extraordinary person revealed.

Unlike other psychologists who have done research on people with an exceptional gift for
memory, the author did not confine himself to meas-
uring the capacity and stability of the subject's memory, or to describing the devices used by the latter
to recall and reproduce material. He was far more
interested in studying certain other issues: What
effect does a remarkable capacity for memory have
on other major aspects of personality, on an individual's habits of thought and imagination, on his
behavior and personality development? What
changes occur in a person's inner world, in his relationships with others, in his very life style when
one element of his psychic makeup, his memory,
develops to such an uncommon degree that it begins
to alter every other aspect of his activity?

Such an approach to the study of psychic phenomena is hardly typical of scientific psychology,
which deals for the most part with sensation and
perception, attention and memory, thinking and
emotion, but only rarely considers how the entire
structure of an individual's personality may hinge
on the development of one of these features of
psychic activity.

Nonetheless, this approach has been in use for
some time. It is the accepted method in clinical
medicine, where the thoughtful physician is never
interested merely in the course of a disease he hap-

pens to be studying at the moment, but tries to determine what effect a disturbance of one particular process has on other organic processes; how changes in the latter (which ultimately have one root cause) alter the activity of the entire organism, thus giving rise to the total *picture of disease,* to what medicine commonly terms a *syndrome.*

The study of syndromes, however, need not be restricted to clinical medicine. By the same token, one can analyze how an unusually developed feature of psychic makeup produces changes, which are causally related to it, in the entire structure of psychic life, in the total personality. In the latter instance, too, we would be dealing with "syndromes" having one causal factor, except that these would be psychological rather than clinical syndromes.

It is precisely with the emergence of such a syndrome, one produced by an exceptional memory, that this book is concerned. The author hopes that by reading it psychologists may be prompted to investigate and describe other psychological syndromes: the distinct personality features which emerge when there is heightened development of an individual's sensitivity or imagination, his power of observation or capacity for abstract thought, or the will power he exerts in the pursuit of a particular idea. This would mark the beginning of a concrete (but nonetheless scientifically valid) psychology.

That an analysis of an exceptional memory, of the role it played in shaping an individual's psychic makeup, should initiate this type of research has certain distinct advantages. Memory studies, which had been at a standstill for so many years, have once again become a subject of vital research, leading to rapid growth in our knowledge of this particular phenomenon. This progress is bound up with the development of a new branch of technology, bionics, which has forced us to take a closer look at every possible indication of how the human memory operates: the devices it uses as a basis for the mental "notes" people take on their impressions of things; the "readings" the mind takes of memory traces that have been retained. At the same time, recent work on memory is related to advances in our knowledge made possible through current theories of the brain, its physiological and biochemical structure.

Nevertheless, in this book we will not be drawing either on information acquired in these fields or on the vast literature available on memory. This book is devoted to the study of *one man,* and the author will venture no further than what observations on this remarkable "experiment of nature" themselves provided.

# 2

## *The Beginning of the Research*

The actual beginning of this account dates back to the 1920's, when I had only recently begun to do work in psychology. It was then that a man came to my laboratory who asked me to test his memory.

At the time the man (let us designate him S.) was a newspaper reporter who had come to my laboratory at the suggestion of the paper's editor. Each morning the editor would meet with the staff and hand out assignments for the day—lists of places he wanted covered, information to be obtained in each. The list of addresses and instructions was usually fairly long, and the editor noted with some surprise that S. never took any notes.

He was about to reproach the reporter for being inattentive when, at his urging, S. repeated the entire assignment word for word. Curious to learn more about how the man operated, the editor began questioning S. about his memory. But S. merely countered with amazement: Was there really anything unusual about his remembering everything he'd been told? Wasn't that the way other people operated? The idea that he possessed certain particular qualities of memory which distinguished him from others struck him as incomprehensible.

The editor sent him to the psychology laboratory to have some studies done on his memory, and thus it was that I found myself confronted with the man.

At the time S. was just under thirty. The information I got on his family background was that his father owned a bookstore, that his mother, an elderly Jewish woman, was quite well-read, and that of his numerous brothers and sisters (all of them conventional, well-balanced types) some were gifted individuals. There was no incidence of mental illness in the family.

S. had grown up in a small Jewish community and had attended elementary school there. Later, when it was discovered that he had musical ability, he was enrolled in a music school, where he studied in the hope that he might some day become a professional violinist. However, after an ear disease had left his hearing somewhat impaired, he realized he could hardly expect to have a successful career as a musician. During the time he spent looking for the sort of work that would best suit him he happened to visit the newspaper, where he subsequently began work as a reporter.

S. had no clear idea what he wanted out of life, and his plans were fairly indefinite. The impression he gave was of a rather ponderous and at times timid person who was puzzled at having been sent to the psychology laboratory. As I mentioned, he wasn't aware of any peculiarities in himself and couldn't conceive of the idea that his memory differed in some way from other people's. He passed on his editor's request to me with some degree of confusion and waited curiously to see what, if anything, the research might turn up. Thus began a relationship of almost thirty years, filled with experiments, discussions, and correspondence.

When I began my study of S. it was with much the same degree of curiosity psychologists generally have at the outset of research, hardly with the hope that the experiments would offer anything of particular note. However, the results of the first tests were enough to change my attitude and to leave me, the experimenter, rather than my subject, both embarrassed and perplexed.

I gave S. a series of words, then numbers, then

letters, reading them to him slowly or presenting them in written form. He read or listened attentively and then repeated the material exactly as it had been presented. I increased the number of elements in each series, giving him as many as thirty, fifty, or even seventy words or numbers, but this, too, presented no problem for him. He did not need to commit any of the material to memory; if I gave him a series of words or numbers, which I read slowly and distinctly, he would listen attentively, sometimes ask me to stop and enunciate a word more clearly, or, if in doubt whether he had heard a word correctly, would ask me to repeat it. Usually during an experiment he would close his eyes or stare into space, fixing his gaze on one point; when the experiment was over, he would ask that we pause while he went over the material in his mind to see if he had retained it. Thereupon, without another moment's pause, he would reproduce the series that had been read to him.

The experiment indicated that he could reproduce a series in reverse order—from the end to the beginning—just as simply as from start to finish; that he could readily tell me which word followed another in a series, or reproduce the word which happened to precede one I'd name. He would pause for a minute, as though searching for the word, but immediately after would be able to answer my questions and generally made no mistakes.

It was of no consequence to him whether the series I gave him contained meaningful words or nonsense syllables, numbers or sounds; whether they were presented orally or in writing. All he required was that there be a three-to-four-second pause between each element in the series, and he had no difficulty reproducing whatever I gave him.

As the experimenter, I soon found myself in a state verging on utter confusion. An increase in the length of a series led to no noticeable increase in difficulty for S., and I simply had to admit that the capacity of his memory *had no distinct limits;* that I had been unable to perform what one would think was the simplest task a psychologist can do: measure the capacity of an individual's memory. I arranged a second and then a third session with S.; these were followed by a series of sessions, some of them days and weeks apart, others separated by a period of several years.

But these later sessions only further complicated my position as experimenter, for it appeared that there was no limit either to the *capacity* of S.'s memory or to the *durability of the traces he retained.* Experiments indicated that he had no difficulty reproducing any lengthy series of words whatever, even though these had originally been presented to him a week, a month, a year, or even many years earlier. In fact, some of these experiments designed to test his retention were performed (without his being given any warning) fifteen or sixteen years after the session in which he had originally recalled the words. Yet invariably they were successful. During these test sessions S. would sit with his eyes closed, pause, then comment: "Yes, yes . . . This was a series you gave me once when we were in your apartment . . . You were sitting at the table and I in the rocking chair . . . You were wearing a gray suit and you looked at me like this . . . Now, then, I can see you saying . . ." And with that he would reel off the series precisely as I had given it to him at the earlier session. If one takes into account that S. had by then become a well-known mnemonist, who had to remember hundreds and thousands of series, the feat seems even more remarkable.

All this meant that I had to alter my plan and concentrate less on any attempt to *measure* the man's memory than on some way to provide a *qualitative analysis* of it, to describe the *psychological aspects of its structure.* Subsequently I undertook to explore another problem, as I said, to do a close study of the peculiarities that seemed an inherent part of the psychology of this exceptional mnemonist.

I devoted the balance of my research to these two tasks, the results of which I will try to present systematically here, though many years have passed since my work with S.

# 3

## *His Memory*

This study of S.'s memory was begun in the mid-1920's, when he was still working as a newspaper reporter. It continued for many years, during which S. changed jobs several times, finally becoming a professional mnemonist who gave performances of memory feats. Although the procedures S. used to recall material retained their original pattern throughout this time, they gradually became enriched with new devices, so that ultimately they presented quite a different picture psychologically.

In this section we will consider the peculiar features his memory exhibited at successive stages.

### THE INITIAL FACTS

Throughout the course of our research S.'s recall was always of a spontaneous nature. The only mechanisms he employed were one of the following: either he continued to *see* series of words or numbers which had been presented to him, or he converted these elements into *visual images*.

The simplest structure was one S. used to recall *tables of numbers* written on a blackboard. S. would study the material on the board, close his eyes, open them again for a moment, turn aside, and, at a signal, reproduce one series from the board. Then he would fill in the empty squares of the next table, rapidly calling off the numbers. It was a simple matter for him to fill in the numbers for the empty squares of the table either when asked to do this for certain squares I chose at random, or when asked to fill in a series of numbers successively in reverse order. He could easily tell me which numbers formed one or another of the vertical columns in the table and could "read off" to me numbers that formed the diagonals; finally, he was able to compose a multi-digit number out of the one-digit numbers in the entire table.

In order to imprint an impression of a table consisting of twenty numbers, S. needed only 35–40 seconds, during which he would examine the chart closely several times. A table of fifty numbers required somewhat more time, but he could easily fix an impression of it in his mind in 2.5–3 minutes, staring at the chart a few times, then closing his eyes as he tested himself on the material in his mind.

The following is a typical example of one of dozens of experiments that were carried out with him (Experiment of May 10, 1939):

TABLE 1

| | | | |
|---|---|---|---|
| 6 | 6 | 8 | 0 |
| 5 | 4 | 3 | 2 |
| 1 | 6 | 8 | 4 |
| 7 | 9 | 3 | 5 |
| 4 | 2 | 3 | 7 |
| 3 | 8 | 9 | 1 |
| 1 | 0 | 0 | 2 |
| 3 | 4 | 5 | 1 |
| 2 | 7 | 6 | 8 |
| 1 | 9 | 2 | 6 |
| 2 | 9 | 6 | 7 |
| 5 | 5 | 2 | 0 |
| x | 0 | 1 | x |

He spent three minutes examining the table I had drawn on a piece of paper (Table 1), stopping intermittently to go over what he had seen in his mind. It took him 40 seconds to reproduce this table (that is, to call off all the numbers in succession). He did this at a rhythmic pace, scarcely pausing between numbers. His reproduction of the numbers in the third vertical column took somewhat longer—1 minute, 20 seconds—whereas he reproduced those in the second vertical column in 25 seconds, and took 30 seconds to reproduce this column in reverse order. He read off the numbers which formed the diagonals (the groups of four numbers running zigzag through the chart) in 35 seconds, and within 50 seconds ran through the numbers that formed the horizontal rows. Altogether he required 1 minute, 30 seconds to convert all fifty numbers into a single fifty-digit number and read this off.

As I have already mentioned, an experiment designed to verify S.'s "reading" of this series, which was not carried out until after several months had elapsed, indicated that he could reproduce the table he had "impressed" in his mind just as fully as in the first reproduction and at about the same rates. The only difference in the two performances was that for the later one he needed more time to "revive" the entire situation in which the experiment had originally been carried out: to "see" the room in which we had been sitting; to "hear" my voice;

to "reproduce" an image of himself looking at the board. But the actual process of "reading" the table required scarcely any more time than it had earlier.

Similar data were obtained in experiments in which we presented S. with a table of letters written either on a blackboard or on a sheet of paper. It took him roughly the same amount of time both to register an impression of these meaningless series of letters and to read them off as he had needed for the table of numbers. (See Table 2: experimental material given S. during a session at which the academician L. A. Orbeli was present.) S. reproduced this material with the same ease he had demonstrated earlier, there being no distinct limits, apparently, either to the capacity of his memory or to the stability of the impressions he formed.

TABLE 2

| ZH* | CH* | SH* | T | I | P | R |
|-----|-----|-----|---|---|-----|-----|
| K | P | O | S | M | K | SH* |
| L | T | O | A | L | KH* | T |
| M | T | ZH* | S | K | R | CH* |
| etc. | | | | | | |

\* In Russian, single letters: ZH = Ж, CH = Ч, SH = Ш, KH = Х.

But precisely how did he manage to register an "imprint" and "read off" the tables he had been shown? The only possible way to determine this was to question S. himself.

At first glance the explanation seems quite simple. He told us that he continued *to see* the table which had been written on a blackboard or a sheet of paper, that he merely had to "read it off," successively enumerating the numbers or letters it contained. Hence, it generally made no difference to him whether he "read" the table from the beginning or the end, whether he listed the elements that formed the vertical or the diagonal groups, or "read off" numbers that formed the horizontal rows. The task of converting the individual numbers into a single, multi-digit number appeared to be no more difficult for him than it would be for others of us were we asked to perform this operation visually and given a considerably longer time to study the table.

S. continued to see the numbers he had "imprinted" in his memory just as they had appeared on the board or the sheet of paper: the numbers presented exactly the same configuration they had as written, so that if one of the numbers had not been written distinctly, S. was liable to "misread" it, to take a 3 for an 8, for example, or a 4 for a 9. However, even at this stage of the report our attention had been drawn to certain peculiarities in S.'s account which indicated that his process of recall was not at all simple.

## SYNESTHESIA

Our curiosity had been aroused by a small and seemingly unimportant observation. S. had remarked on a number of occasions that if the examiner said something during the experiment—if, for example, he said "yes" to confirm that S. had reproduced the material correctly or "no" to indicate he had made a mistake—a blur would appear on the table and would spread and block off the numbers, so that S. in his mind would be forced to "shift" the table over, away from the blurred section that was covering it. The same thing happened if he heard noise in the auditorium; this was immediately converted into "puffs of steam" or "splashes" which made it more difficult for him to read the table.

This led us to believe that the process by which he retained material did not consist merely of his having preserved spontaneous traces of visual impressions; there were certain additional elements at work. I suggested that S. possessed a marked degree of *synesthesia*. If we can trust S.'s recollections of his early childhood (which we will deal with in a special section later in this account), these synesthetic reactions could be traced back to a very early age. As he described it:

When I was about two or three years old I was taught the words of a Hebrew prayer. I didn't understand them, and what happened was that the words settled in my mind as puffs of steam or splashes . . . Even now I *see* these puffs or splashes when I hear certain sounds.

Synesthetic reactions of this type occurred whenever S. was asked to listen to *tones*. The same reactions, though somewhat more complicated, occurred with his perception of *voices* and with speech sounds.

The following is the record of experiments that were carried out with S. in the Laboratory on the Physiology of Hearing at the Neurological Institute, Academy of Medical Sciences.

Presented with a tone pitched at 30 cycles per second and having an amplitude of 100 decibels, S. stated that at first he saw a strip 12–15 cm. in width the color of old, tarnished silver. Gradually this strip narrowed and seemed to recede; then it was converted into an object that glistened like steel. Then the tone gradually took on a color one associates with twilight, the sound continuing to dazzle because of the silvery gleam it shed.

Presented with a tone pitched at 50 cycles per second and an amplitude of 100 decibels, S. saw a brown strip against a dark background that had red, tongue-like edges. The sense of taste he experienced was like that of sweet and sour borscht, a sensation that gripped his entire tongue.

Presented with a tone pitched at 100 cycles per second and having an amplitude of 86 decibels, he saw a wide strip that appeared to have a reddish-orange hue in the center; from the center outwards the brightness faded with light gradations so that the edges of the strip appeared pink.

Presented with a tone pitched at 250 cycles per second and having an amplitude of 64 decibels, S. saw a velvet cord with fibers jutting out on all sides. The cord was tinged with a delicate, pleasant pink-orange hue.

Presented with a tone pitched at 500 cycles per second and having an amplitude of 100 decibels, he saw a streak of lightning splitting the heavens in two. When the intensity of the sound was lowered to 74 decibels, he saw a dense orange color which made him feel as though a needle had been thrust into his spine. Gradually this sensation diminished.

Presented with a tone pitched at 2,000 cycles per second and having an amplitude of 113 decibels, S. said: "It looks something like fireworks tinged with a pink-red hue. The strip of color feels rough and unpleasant, and it has an ugly taste—rather like that of a briny pickle . . . You could hurt your hand on this."

Presented with a tone pitched at 3,000 cycles per second and having an amplitude of 128 decibels, he saw a whisk broom that was of a fiery color, while the rod attached to the whisks seemed to be scattering off into fiery points.

The experiments were repeated during several days and invariably the same stimuli produced identical experiences.

What this meant was that S. was one of a remarkable group of people, among them the composer Scriabin, who have retained in an especially vivid form a "complex" synesthetic type of sensitivity. In S.'s case every sound he heard immediately produced an experience of light and color and, as we shall see later in this account, a sense of taste and touch as well.

S. also experienced synesthetic reactions when he listened to someone's *voice*. "What a crumbly, yellow voice you have," he once told L. S. Vygotsky* while conversing with him. At a later date he elaborated on the subject of voices as follows:

You know there are people who seem to have many voices, whose voices seem to be an entire composition, a bouquet. The late S. M. Eisenstein† had just such a voice: listening to him, it was as though a flame with fibers protruding from it was advancing right toward me. I got so interested in his voice, I couldn't follow what he was saying . . .

* The well-known Russian psychologist. [Tr.]
† The famous producer. [Tr.]

But there are people whose voices change constantly. I frequently have trouble recognizing someone's voice over the phone, and it isn't merely because of a bad connection. It's because the person happens to be someone whose voice changes twenty to thirty times in the course of a day. Other people don't notice this, but I do.

(Record of November 1951.)

To this day I can't escape from seeing colors when I hear sounds. What first strikes me is the color of someone's voice. Then it fades off . . . for it does interfere. If, say, a person says something, I see the word; but should another person's voice break in, blurs appear. These creep into the syllables of the words and I can't make out what is being said.

(Record of June 1953.)

"Lines," "blurs," and "splashes" would emerge not only when he heard tones, noises, or voices. Every speech sound immediately summoned up for S. a striking visual image, for it had its own distinct form, color, and taste. Vowels appeared to him as simple figures, consonants as splashes, some of them solid configurations, others more scattered —but all of them retained some distinct form. As he described it:

A [a] is something white and long; и [ɛ] moves off somewhere ahead so that you just can't sketch it, whereas й [j'ɪ] is pointed in form. Ю [j'u] is also pointed and sharper than e [j'ɛ], whereas я [j'ɑ] is big, so big that you can actually roll right over it. O [ɔ] is a sound that comes from your chest . . . it's broad, though the sound itself tends to fall. Эй [j'ɔ] moves off somewhere to the side. I also experience a sense of taste from each sound. And when I see lines, some configuration that has been drawn, these produce sounds. Take the figure ⌐____. This is somewhere in between e, Ю, and И; ᵚᵚᵚᵚ is a vowel sound, but it also resembles the sound r—not a pure r though . . . But one thing still isn't clear to me: if the line goes up, I experience a sound, but if it moves in the reverse direction, it no longer comes through as a sound but as some sort of wooden hook for a yoke. The configuration ⌣ʄ appears to be something dark, but if it had been drawn slower, it would have seemed different. Had you, say, drawn it like this ⌣ʄ′, then it would have been the sound e.

## S. had similar experiences with numbers:

For me 2, 4, 6, 5 are not just numbers. They have forms. 1 is a pointed number—which has nothing to do with the way it's written. It's because it's somehow firm and complete. 2 is flatter, rectangular, whitish in color, sometimes almost a gray. 3 is a pointed segment which rotates. 4 is also square and dull; it looks like 2 but has more substance to it, it's thicker. 5 is absolutely complete and takes the form of a cone or a tower—something substantial. 6, the first number after 5, has a whitish hue; 8 somehow has a naïve quality, it's milky blue like lime . . .

What this indicates is that for S. there was no distinct line, as there is for others of us, separating vision from hearing, or hearing from a sense of touch or taste. The remnants of synesthesia that many ordinary people have, which are of a very rudimentary sort (experiencing lower and higher tones as having different colorations; regarding some tones as "warm," others as "cold"; "seeing" Friday and Monday as having different colors), were central to S.'s psychic life. These synesthetic experiences not only appeared very early in his life but persisted right to his death. And, as we shall have occasion to see, they left their mark on his habits of perception, understanding, and thought, and were a vital feature of his memory.

S.'s tendency to recall material in terms of "lines" or "splashes" came into play whenever he had to deal with isolated sounds, nonsense syllables, or words he was not familiar with. He pointed out that in these circumstances sounds, voices, or words evoked some visual impression such as "puffs of steam," "splashes," "smooth or broken lines"; sometimes they also produced a sensation of taste, at other times a sensation of touch, of his having come into contact with something he would describe as "prickly," "smooth," or "rough."

These synesthetic components of each visual and particularly of each auditory stimulus had been an inherent part of S.'s recall at a very early age; it was only later, after his faculty for logical and figurative memory had developed, that these tended to fade into the background, though they continued to play some part in his recall.

From an objective standpoint these synesthetic components were important to his recall, for they created, as it were, a background for each recollection, furnishing him with additional, "extra" information that would guarantee accurate recall. If, as we shall see later, S. was prompted to reproduce a word inaccurately, the additional synesthetic sensations he experienced would fail to coincide with the word he produced, leaving him with the sense that something was wrong with his response and forcing him to correct the error.

... I recognize a word not only by the images it evokes but by a whole complex of feelings that image arouses. It's hard to express ... it's not a matter of vision or hearing but some over-all sense I get. Usually I experience a word's taste and weight, and I don't have to make an effort to remember it—the word seems to recall itself. But it's difficult to describe. What I sense is something oily slipping through my hand ... or I'm aware of a slight tickling in my left hand caused by a mass of tiny, lightweight points. When that happens I simply remember, without having to make the attempt ...

(Record of May 22, 1939.)

Hence, the synesthetic experiences that clearly made themselves felt when he recalled a voice, individual sounds, or complexes of sound were not of major importance but served merely as information that was secondary in *his recall of words*. Let us consider S.'s responses to words now in greater detail.

## WORDS AND IMAGES

As we know, there are two aspects to the nature of words. On the one hand, words are composed of conventional groupings of *sounds* having various degrees of complexity—the feature of language phonetics deals with. On the other hand, words also designate certain objects, qualities, or activities; that is, they have specific *meanings*—that aspect of words with which semantics and other related branches of linguistics, such as lexicology and morphology, are concerned. A person in a healthy, alert state of awareness will generally not notice the phonetic elements in words, so that given two words such as *skripka* and *skrepka* (Russian: "violin" and "paper clip"), which differ by virtue of one minor alteration of vowel sounds, he may be completely unaware of their resemblance phonetically and observe only that they stand for two completely different things.*

For S., too, it was the meaning of words that was predominantly important. Each word had the effect of summoning up in his mind a graphic image, and what distinguished him from the general run of people was that his images were incomparably more vivid and stable than theirs. Further, his images were invariably linked with synesthetic components (sensations of colored "splotches," "splashes," and "lines") which reflected the sound structure of a word and the voice of the speaker.

It was only natural, then, that the *visual quality of his recall* was fundamental to his capacity for remembering words. For when he heard or read a word it was at once converted into a visual image corresponding with the object the word signified for him. Once he formed an image, which was always of a particularly vivid nature, it stabilized itself in his memory, and though it might vanish for a time when his attention was taken up with something else, it would manifest itself once again whenever he returned to the situation in which the word had first come up. As he described it:

* It is only in certain pathological states that the phonetic elements of words predominate and meaning becomes unimportant. See A. R. Luria and O. S. Vinogradova: "An Objective Investigation of the Dynamics of Semantic Systems," *British Journal of Psychology*, L, No. 2 (1959), 89–105.

When I hear the word *green,* a green flowerpot appears; with the word *red* I see a man in a red shirt coming toward me; as for *blue,* this means an image of someone waving a small blue flag from a window . . . Even numbers remind me of images. Take the number 1. This is a proud, well-built man; 2 is a high-spirited woman; 3 a gloomy person (why, I don't know); 6 a man with a swollen foot; 7 a man with a mustache; 8 a very stout woman—a sack within a sack. As for the number 87, what I see is a fat woman and a man twirling his mustache.

(Record of September 1936.)

One can easily see that the images produced by numbers and words represent a fusion of graphic ideas and synesthetic reactions. If S. heard a word he was familiar with, the image would be sufficient to screen off any synesthetic reactions; but if he had to deal with an unfamiliar word, which did not evoke an image, he would remember it "in terms of lines." In other words, the sounds of the word were transformed into colored splotches, lines, or splashes. Thus, even with an unfamiliar word, he still registered some visual impression which he associated with it but which was related to the phonetic qualities of the word rather than to its meaning.

When S. read through a long series of words, each word would elicit a graphic image. And since the series was fairly long, he had to find some way of distributing these images of his in a mental row or sequence. Most often (and this habit persisted throughout his life), he would "distribute" them along some roadway or street he visualized in his mind. Sometimes this was a street in his home town, which would also include the yard attached to the house he had lived in as a child and which he recalled vividly. On the other hand, he might also select a street in Moscow. Frequently he would take a mental walk along that street—Gorky Street in Moscow—beginning at Mayakovsky Square, and slowly make his way down, "distributing" his images at houses, gates, and store windows. At times, without realizing how it had happened, he would suddenly find himself back in his home town (Torzhok), where he would wind up his trip in the house he had lived in as a child. The setting he chose for his "mental walks" approximates that of dreams, the difference being that the setting in his walks would immediately vanish once his attention was distracted but would reappear just as suddenly when he was obliged to recall a series he had "recorded" this way.

This technique of converting a series of words into a series of graphic images explains why S. could so readily reproduce a series from start to finish or in reverse order; how he could rapidly name the word that preceded or followed one I'd select from the series. To do this, he would simply begin his walk, either from the beginning or from the end of the street, find the image of the object I had named, and "take a look at" whatever happened to be situated on either side of it. S.'s visual patterns of memory differed from the more commonplace type of figurative memory by virtue of the fact that his images were exceptionally vivid and stable; he was also able to "turn away" from them, as it were, and "return" to them whenever it was necessary.*

It was this technique of recalling material graphically that explained why S. always insisted a series be read clearly and distinctly, that the words not be read off too quickly. For he needed some time, however slight, to convert the words into images. If the words were read too quickly, without sufficient pause between them, his images would tend to coalesce into a kind of chaos or "noise" through which he had difficulty discerning anything.

In effect, the astonishing clarity and tenacity of his images, the fact that he could retain them for years and call them up when occasion demanded it,

---

* S.'s technique of a "graphic distribution" and "reading" of images closely resembled that of another mnemonist, Ishihara, who was studied and written about in Japan. See Tukasa Susukita: "Untersuchung eines ausserordentlichen Gedächtnisses," *Japan Tohoku Psychologica Folia,* I, No. 2–3, and II, No. 1, Tohoky Imperialis Universitas, Sendai, 1933.

made it possible for him to recall an unlimited number of words and to retain these indefinitely. Nonetheless, his method of "recording" also had certain drawbacks.

Once we were convinced that the capacity of S.'s memory was virtually unlimited, that he did not have to "memorize" the data presented but merely had to "register an impression," which he could "read" on a much later date (in this account we will cite instances of series he reproduced ten or even sixteen years after the original presentation), we naturally lost interest in trying to "measure" his memory capacity. Instead, we concentrated on precisely the reverse issue: Was it possible for him to forget? We tried to establish the instances in which S. had omitted a word from a series.

Indeed, not only were such instances to be found, but they were fairly frequent. Yet how was one to explain forgetting in a man whose memory seemed inexhaustible? How explain that sometimes there were instances in which S. *omitted* some elements in his recall but scarcely ever *reproduced material inaccurately* (by substituting a synonym or a word closely associated in meaning with the one he'd been given)?

The experiments immediately turned up answers to both questions. S. did not "forget" words he'd been given; what happened was that he omitted these as he "read off" a series. And in each case there was a simple explanation for the omissions. If S. had placed a particular image in a spot where it would be difficult for him to "discern"—if he, for example, had placed it in an area that was poorly lit or in a spot where he would have trouble distinguishing the object from the background against which it had been set—he would omit this image when he "read off" the series he had distributed along his mental route. He would simply walk on "without noticing" the particular item, as he explained.

These omissions (and they were quite frequent in the early period of our observation, when S.'s technique of recall had not developed to its fullest) clearly were not *defects of memory* but were, in fact, *defects of perception*. They could not be explained in terms of established ideas on the neurodynamics of memory traces (retroactive and proactive inhibition, extinction of traces, etc.) but rather by certain factors that influence perception (clarity, contrast, the ability to isolate a figure from its background, the degree of lighting available, etc.). His errors could not be explained, then, in terms of the psychology of memory but had to do with the psychological factors that govern perception.

Excerpts from the numerous reports taken on

our sessions with S. will serve to illustrate this point. When, for example, S. reproduced a long series of words, he omitted the word *pencil;* on another occasion he skipped *egg;* in a third series it was the word *banner,* and in a fourth, *blimp.* Finally, S. omitted from another series the word *shuttle,* which he was not familiar with. The following is his explanation of how this happened:

I put the image of the *pencil* near a fence . . . the one down the street, you know. But what happened was that the image fused with that of the fence and I walked right on past without noticing it. The same thing happened with the word *egg.* I had put it up against a white wall and it blended in with the background. How could I possibly spot a white egg up against a white wall? Now take the word *blimp.* That's something gray, so it blended in with the gray of the pavement . . . *Banner,* of course, means the Red Banner. But, you know, the building which houses the Moscow City Soviet of Workers' Deputies is also red, and since I'd put the banner close to one of the walls of the building I just walked on without seeing it . . . Then there's the word *putamen.* I don't know what this means, but it's such a dark word that I couldn't see it . . . and, besides, the street lamp was quite a distance away . . .
(Record of December 1932.)

Sometimes I put a word in a dark place and have trouble seeing it as I go by. Take the word *box,* for example. I'd put it in a niche in the gate. Since it was dark there I couldn't see it . . . Sometimes if there is noise, or another person's voice suddenly intrudes, I see blurs which block off my images. Then syllables are liable to slip into a word which weren't there originally and I'd be tempted to say they really had been part of the word. It's these blurs which interfere with my recall . . .

(Record of December 1932.)

Hence, S.'s "defects of memory" were really "defects of perception" or "concentration." An analysis of them allowed us to get a better grasp of the characteristic devices this amazing man used to recall words, without altering our former impressions with respect to the power of his memory. Upon closer examination, these devices also provided an answer to our second question: Why was it that S. evidenced no distortions of memory?

This last could be explained simply in terms of the synesthetic components that entered into his "recording" and "reading" of memory traces. As mentioned earlier, S. did not just transcribe words he had been given into graphic images: each word also furnished him with "extra" information which took the form of synesthetic impressions of sight, taste, and touch, all of these aroused either by the sound of a word or by images of the letters in the written word. If S. made a mistake when he "read off" his images, the extra information he had also registered would not coincide with the other characteristics of the word he had reproduced (a synonym, perhaps, or a word closely associated in meaning with the correct word). He would then be left with some sense of disharmony that would alert him to his mistake.

I remember once walking back with S. from the institute where we had been conducting some experiments with L. A. Orbeli. "You won't forget the way back to the institute?" I asked, forgetting whom I was dealing with. "Come, now," S. said. "How could I possibly forget? After all, here's this fence. It has such a salty taste and feels so rough; furthermore, it has such a sharp, piercing sound . . ."

The combination of various indications which, owing to S.'s synesthetic experiences, provided him with additional information on each impression he had registered operated to guarantee that his recall would be precise, or made it highly unlikely that he would come up with a response that would differ from the word he had been given.

### DIFFICULTIES

Despite the advantages S. derived from having spontaneous visual recall, his was a type of memory that had certain drawbacks as well, a fact which became all the more apparent when he was forced to remember a greater quantity of material that was constantly subject to change. This was a problem he was often faced with after he quit his newspaper job and became a professional mnemonist.

We have already dealt with the first type of difficulty, that related to perception. Once S. had begun his career as a mnemonist, he could no longer reconcile himself to the possibility that individual images might merge with the background setting or that he might have trouble "reading" them off because of "bad lighting." Nor could he accept as a matter of course the idea that noise could produce "blurs," "splashes," or "puffs of steam" that would block off the images he had distributed, making it difficult to "single them out." As he put it:

You see, every sound bothers me . . . it's transformed into a line and becomes confusing. Once I had the word *omnia*. It got entangled in noise and I recorded *omnion*. . . . sometimes I find that instead of the word I have to turn up I see lines of some sort . . . But I touch them, and somehow they're worn away by the touch of my hands . . . Other times smoke or fog appears . . . and the more people talk, the harder it gets, until I reach a point where I can't make anything out . . .

(Record of May 1935.)

It often happened, too, that he would be given words to remember which ranged so far in meaning that his system of "distributing" the corresponding images for these words would break down.

I had just started out from Mayakovsky Square when they gave me the word *Kremlin,* so I had to get myself off to the Kremlin. Okay, I can throw a rope across to it . . . But right after that they gave me the word *poetry* and once again I found myself on Pushkin Square. If I'd been given *American Indian,* I'd have had to get to America. I could, of course, throw a rope across the ocean, but it's so exhausting traveling . . .

(Record of May 1935.)

His situation was even further complicated by the fact that the spectators at his demonstrations would deliberately give him long, confusing, or even senseless words to remember. This led him to try to remember these "in terms of lines." But then he had to visualize all the curves, colors, and splashes into which the sounds of a voice were transformed, a difficult job to handle. He realized that his graphic, figurative type of memory did not operate in sufficiently economical ways to allow for such a volume of material, that he had to find some means of adapting it to the demands his work made on him.

This marked the beginning of a second stage of development in which S. tried both to simplify his manner of recall and to devise a new method that would enrich his memory and make it less vulnerable to chance; a method, in short, that would guarantee rapid, precise recall of any type of material, regardless of circumstances.

## EIDOTECHNIQUE (TECHNIQUE OF EIDETIC IMAGES)

The first step was to eliminate the possibility of any chance circumstance that might make it difficult for him to "read" his images when he wished to recall material. This proved quite simple.

I know that I have to be on guard if I'm not to overlook something. What I do now is to make my images larger. Take the word *egg* I told you about before. It was so easy to lose sight of it; now I make it a larger image, and when I lean it up against the wall of a building, I see to it that the place is lit up by having a street lamp nearby . . . I don't put things in dark passageways any more . . . Much better if there's some light around, it's easier to spot then.

(Record of June 1935.)

Increasing the dimensions of his images, seeing to it that the images were clearly illuminated and suitably arranged—this marked the first step in S.'s technique of eidetic images, which described the second phase of his memory development. Another device he developed was a shorthand system for his images, of providing abbreviated or symbolic versions of them. He had not attempted this technique during his early development, but in time it became one of the principal methods he used in his work as a professional mnemonist. This is the description he gave us:

Formerly, in order to remember a thing, I would have to summon up an image of the whole scene. Now all I have to do is take some detail I've decided on in advance that will signify the whole image. Say I'm given the word *horseman*. All it takes now is an image of a foot in a spur. Earlier, if I'd been given the word *restaurant,* I'd have seen the entrance to the restaurant, people sitting inside, a Rumanian orchestra tuning up, and a lot else . . . Now if I'm given the word, I'd see something rather like a store and an entranceway with a bit of something white showing from inside—that's all, and I'd remember the word. So my images have changed quite a bit. Earlier they were more clear-cut, more realistic. The ones I have now are not as well defined or as vivid as the earlier ones . . . I try just to single out one detail I'll need in order to remember a word.

(Record of December 1935.)

The course his technique of using eidetic images took, then, was to abbreviate images and abstract from them the vital details that would allow him to generalize to the whole. He worked out a similar method whereby he could eliminate the need for any detailed, intricate images.

Earlier, if I were to remember the word *America,* I'd have had to stretch a long, long rope across the ocean, from Gorky Street to America, so as not to lose the way. This isn't necessary any more. Say I'm given the word *elephant:* I'd see a zoo. If they gave me *America,* I'd set up an image of Uncle Sam; if *Bismarck,* I'd place my image near the statue of Bismarck; and if I had the word *transcendent,* I'd see my teacher Sherbiny standing and looking at a monument . . . I don't go through all those complicated operations any more, getting myself to different countries in order to remember words.

(Record of May 1935.)

By abbreviating his images, finding symbolic forms for them, S. soon came to a third device that proved to be central to his system of recall.

Since he had thousands of words to deal with in performances—often, words his audience made deliberately complicated and meaningless—S. was forced to *convert senseless words into intelligible images.* He found that the fastest way to do this was to break the words or meaningless phrases down into their component parts and try to attach meaning to an individual syllable by linking it up with some association. This technique required training, but in time, working at it several hours a day, S. became a virtuoso at breaking down senseless elements of words or phrases into intelligible parts which he could automatically convert into images. Central to this device, which he used with astonishing ease and rapidity, was a process whereby he "semanticized" images, basing them on sounds; in addition, he put to use complexes of synesthetic reactions which, as before, served to guarantee him accurate recall. Note his description of the technique:

If, say, I'm given a phrase I don't understand, such as *Ibi bene ubi patria,* I'd have an image of Benya (*bene*) and his father (*pater*). I'd simply have to remember that they're off in the woods somewhere in a little house having an argument . . .

(Record of December 1932.)

We will limit ourselves to a few examples that should illustrate the virtuosity with which S. employed this technique of combining semantization and eidetic images to remember the following kinds of material: (1) words in a foreign language; (2) a meaningless mathematical formula; and (3) nonsense syllables (the type of material he found most difficult to handle). Interestingly, too, he was able to write these detailed accounts of his performances many years after they had taken place, though he had been given no warning from us, of course, that we would ask for these specific instances of recall.

1. In December 1937, S., who had no knowledge of Italian, was read the first four lines of *The Divine Comedy:*

> Nel mezzo del cammin di nostra vita
> Mi ritrovai per una selva oscura
> Che la diritta via era smarrita
> Ah quanto a dir qual era è cosa dura . . .

As always, S. asked that the words in each line be pronounced distinctly, with slight pauses between words—his one requirement for converting meaningless sound combinations into comprehensible images. And, of course, he was able to use his technique and reproduce several stanzas of *The Divine Comedy,* not only with perfect accuracy of recall, but with the exact stress and pronunciation. Moreover, the test session took place fifteen years after he had memorized these stanzas; and, as usual, he was not forewarned about it.

The following is his account of the methods he used to implement his recall.

[*First line*]
(*Nel*)—I was paying my membership dues when there, in the corridor, I caught sight of the ballerina Nel'skaya.
(*mezzo*)—I myself am a violinist; what I do is to set up an image of a man, together with [Russian: *vmeste*] Nel'skaya, who is playing the violin.

(*del*)—There's a pack of Deli Cigarettes near them.

(*cammin*)—I set up an image of a fireplace [Russian: *kamin*] close by.

(*di*)—Then I see a hand pointing toward a door [Russian: *dver*].

(*nostra*)—I see a nose [Russian: *nos*]; a man has tripped and, in falling, gotten his nose pinched in the doorway (*tra*).

(*vita*)—He lifts his leg over the threshold, for a child is lying there, that is, a sign of life—vitalism.

[*Second line*]

(*Mi*)—Here I set up an image of a Jew who comes out with the remark: "We had nothing to do with it."*

(*ritrovai*): (*ri*)—This is some reply to him on the phone.

(*tru-*)—But since the receiver [Russian: *trubka*] is transparent, it disappears.

(*vai*)—What I see then is an old Jewish woman running off screaming "*Vai!*"

(*per*)—I see her father [*per*] driving along in a cab near the corner of Lubyanka.

(*una*)—But there on the corner of Sukharevka I see a policeman on duty, his bearing so stiff he looks like the figure 1.

(*selva*)—I set up a platform next to him on which Silva is dancing. But just to make sure I won't make a mistake and think this is Silva, I have the stage

* He evokes an image of a Jew whose Yiddish accent alters the pronunciation of the Russian *mwi* ("we"), rendering it "mi." [Tr.]

boards under the platform crack (which gives me the sound *e*).

(*oscura*)—I see a shaft [Russian: *os*] jutting out from the platform pointing in the direction of a hen [Russian: *kuritsa*].

[*Third line*]

(*Che*)—This might be a Chinaman: *cha, chen.**

(*la*)—Next to him I set up an image of his wife, a Parisian.

(*diritta*)—This turns out to be my assistant Margarita.

(*via*)—It is she who says "*via*" [Russian: *vasha,* "your"] and holds out her hand to me.

(*era*)—Really, the things that can happen to a man in this life; he lives a whole "era."

(*smarrita*):(*sma*)—I see a streetcar, a bottle of champagne next to the driver. Behind him sits a Jew wearing a tallith and reciting the *Shmah Israel;* that's where the *sma* comes in. But there's also his daughter (Rita).

[*Fourth line*]

(*Ah*)—*Ahi* in Yiddish means "aha!" So I place a man in the square outside the streetcar who begins to sneeze—*apchkhi!* With this the Yiddish letters *a* and *h* suddenly appear.

(*quanto*)—Here I use a piano with white keys instead of a quint.

(*a dir*)—Here I'm carried back to Torzhok, to my room with the piano, where I see my father-in-law. He says: *Dir!* [Yiddish: "you"]. As for the *a,* I simply

---

* The Italian word *che* had been read incorrectly as having a soft sound. [Tr.]

put an *a* on the table in the room. But since it's a
white sound it's lost in the white of the tablecloth.
(That's why I didn't remember it.)

(*qual era*)—I see a man on horseback, dressed in an
Italian mantle—a cavalier. But just so I won't add
any sounds that weren't in the Italian, I make a
stream of champagne out of my father-in-law's leg:
"Era" Champagne.

(*è*)—This I get out of a line from Gogol: "Who said
'eh'?"—Bobchinsky and Dobchinsky.

(*cosa*)—"It was their servant who saw the goat" [Rus-
sian: *koza*].

(*dura*)—"They said to it: 'What do you think you're
butting into, you fool [Russian: *dura*]?'"

We could go on and quote at length from this
particular record, but the above should suffice to
indicate the methods of recall that S. employed.
One would think a chaotic conglomeration of
images such as this would only complicate the job of
remembering the four lines of the poem. Yet S.
could take these lines, which were written in a
language he did not understand, and in a matter of
minutes compose images that he could "read" off,
thus reproducing the verse exactly as he had
heard it. (And he could manage, also, to repeat
the performance fifteen years later, from memory.)
There can be no doubt that the devices he describes
here were essential to his recall.

2. Toward the end of 1934, S. was asked to

recall a "mathematical" formula that had simply been made up and had no meaning:

$$N \cdot \sqrt{d^2 \times \frac{85}{vx}} \cdot \sqrt[3]{\frac{276^2 \cdot 86x}{n^2 v \cdot \pi 264}} \; n^2 b = sv \; \frac{1624}{32^2} \cdot r^2 s$$

S. examined the formula closely, lifting the paper up several times to get a closer look at it. Then he put it down, shut his eyes for a moment, paused as he "looked the material over" in his mind, and in seven minutes came through with an exact reproduction of the formula. The following account of his indicates the devices he used to aid him in recall.

Neiman ($N$) came out and jabbed at the ground with his cane (.). He looked up at a tall tree which resembled the square-root sign ($\sqrt{\phantom{x}}$), and thought to himself: "No wonder the tree has withered and begun to expose its roots. After all, it was here when I built these two houses" ($d^2$). Once again he poked with his cane (.). Then he said: "The houses are old, I'll have to get rid of them ($\times$);* the sale will bring in far more money." He had originally invested 85,000 in them (85). Then I see the roof of the house detached (———), while down below on the street I see a man playing the Termenvox ($vx$). He's standing near a mailbox, and on the corner there's a large stone (.) which has bccn put there to keep carts from crashing

* The Russian expression literally means to cross out in the sense of "get rid off," to "cross something off one's list." [Tr.]

up against the houses. Here, then, is the square, over there the large tree ($\sqrt{\phantom{x}}$) with three jackdaws on it ($\sqrt[3]{\phantom{x}}$). I simply put the figure 276 here, and a square box containing cigarettes in the "square" ($^2$). The number 86 is written on the box. (This number was also written on the other side of the box, but since I couldn't see it from where I stood I omitted it when I recalled the formula.) As for the $x$, this is a stranger in a black mantle. He is walking toward a fence beyond which is a women's gymnasia. He wants to find some way of getting over the fence (———); he has a rendez-vous with one of the women students ($n$), an elegant young thing who's wearing a gray dress. He's talking as he tries to kick down the boards in the fence with one foot, while with the other ($^2$)—oh, but the girl he runs into turns out to be a different one. She's ugly—phooey! ($v$) . . . At this point I'm carried back to Rezhitsa, to my classroom with the big blackboard . . . I see a cord swinging back and forth there and I put a stop to that (.). On the board I see the figure $\pi264$, and I write after it $n^2b$.

Here I'm back in school. My wife has given me a ruler ($=$). I myself, Solomon-Veniaminovich ($sv$), am sitting there in the class. I see that a friend of mine has written down the figure $\dfrac{1624}{32^2}$. I'm trying to see what else he's written, but behind me are two students, girls ($r^2$), who are also copying and making noise so that he won't notice them. "Sh," I say. "Quiet!" ($s$).

Thus S. managed to reproduce the formula spontaneously, with no errors. Fifteen years later, in 1949, he was still able to trace his pattern of recall in precise detail even though he had had no warning from us that he would be tested on this.

3. In June 1936, S. gave a performance at one of the sanatoria. As he later described it, this was the occasion on which he was given the most difficult material he had ever been asked to memorize. Nonetheless, he not only managed to get through the performance successfully but four years later was able to reproduce it for us.

At the performance, which took place on June 11, 1936, S. was given a long series to recall consisting of nonsense syllables that alternated as follows:

| | | | | | | |
|---|---|---|---|---|---|---|
| 1. | ma | va | na | sa | na | va |
| 2. | na | sa | na | ma | va | |
| 3. | sa | na | ma | va | na | |
| 4. | va | sa | na | va | na | ma |
| 5. | na | va | na | va | sa | ma |
| 6. | na | ma | sa | ma | va | na |
| 7. | sa | ma | sa | va | na | |
| 8. | na | sa | ma | va | ma | na |
| | etc. | | | | | |

S. reproduced the series and four years later, at my request, retraced the method he had used. Following is the description he wrote for us of the performance.

As you remember, in the spring of 1936 I gave a performance which I think is the most difficult I've ever had to give. You had attached a record sheet to the paper and asked that I write down what went on in my mind during that performance when I got through. But since circumstances didn't permit it at the time, it's only now, after four years, that I've finally gotten around to doing this. Even though it's several years since I gave the performance, it's all so vivid, I can see it so clearly, that it seems more like a performance of four months ago, rather than four years ago.

At the performance an assistant read the words off to me, breaking them down into syllables like this: MA VA NA SA NA VA, etc. I'd no sooner heard the first word than I found myself on a road in the forest near the little village of Malta, where my family had had a summer cottage when I was a child. To the left, on a level with my eyes, there appeared an extremely thin line, a grayish-yellow line. This had to do with the fact that all the consonants in the series were coupled with the letter *a*. Then lumps, splashes, blurs, bunches, all of different colors, weights, and thicknesses rapidly appeared on the line; these represented the letters *m, v, n, s,* etc.

The assistant read the second word and at once I saw the same consonants as in the first word, except that they were differently arranged. So I turned left along the road in the forest and continued in a horizontal direction.

The third word. Damn it! The same consonants again, only once again the order has been changed. I asked the assistant whether there were many more words like this, and when he said: "Practically all," I knew I was in for trouble. Realizing I would have this frequent repetition of the same four consonants to deal with, all of them linked to the same monotonous primitive form which the vowel *a* has, was enough to shake my usual confidence. If I was going to have to change paths in the woods for each word, to grope at, smell, and feel each spot, each splash, it might help, but it would take more time. And when you're on stage, each second counts. I could see someone smiling in the audience, and this, too, immediately was converted into an image of a sharp spire, so that I felt as if I'd been stabbed in the heart. I decided to switch to mnemonic techniques that might help me remember the syllables.

Happier now, I asked the assistant to read the first three words again, but this time as a single unit, without breaking them down into syllables. Since the words were nonsensical, the assistant was quite tense as he read them, fearing he would slip up at some point and make a mistake. But the monotonous repetition of the vowel *a* in each syllable helped to create a distinct rhythm and stress, so that the lines sounded like this: MAVÁ—NASÁ—NAVÁ. From this point on, I was able to reproduce the series without pausing, and at a good pace.

This is the way I worked it out in my mind. My landlady (*Mava*), whose house on Slizkaya Street I stayed at while I was in Warsaw, was leaning out of a window that opened onto a courtyard. With her left hand she was pointing inside, toward the room (NASA) [Russian: *nasha,* "our"]; while with her right she was making some negative gesture (NAVA) [Yiddish expression of negation] to a Jew, an old-clothes man, who was standing in the yard with a sack slung over his right shoulder. It was as though she were saying to him: "No, nothing for sale." *Muvi* in Polish means "to speak." As for NASA, I took the Russian *nasha* as its equivalent, remembering all the while that I was substituting a *sh* for the *s* sound in the original word. Further, just as my landlady was saying *"Nasa,"* an orange ray (an image which characterizes the sound *s* for me) suddenly flashed out. As for NAVA, it means "no" in Latvian. The vowels were not important since I knew there was merely the one vowel *a* between all the consonants.

2. NASÁNAMÁVÁ: By this time the old-clothes man had already left the yard and was standing on the street near the gate to the house. Bewildered, he lifted his hands in a gesture of dismay, remembering that the landlady had said we [Russian: *nasha;* that is, NASA] had nothing to sell him. At the same time he was pointing to a full-breasted woman, a wet nurse, who was standing nearby (a wet nurse in Yiddish is *a n'am*). Just then a man who was passing by became indignant with him and said "Vai!" (VA), which is to say, it's shameful for an old Jew to look on at a woman nursing a baby.

3. SANÁMAVÁNÁ: This is where Slizkaya Street begins. I'm standing near the Sukharevaya Tower, approaching it from the direction of First Meshchanskaya Street (for some reason I frequently find myself on this corner during performances). Near the gates to the tower there's a sleigh (SANA) [Russian: *sani*, "sleigh"] in which my landlady (*Mava*) is sitting. She's holding a long white slab with the letters NA [Russian: *na*, "on"] written on it, and on to which the tower is being flung —right through the gates! But where is it heading?

The long slab with the stenciled image NA on, over [Russian: *nad,* "over"] it—higher than any person, higher than a one-story wooden house.

4. VASÁNAVÁNAMÁ: Aha! Here on the corner of Kolkhoznaya Square and Sretenka is the department store where the watchman turns out to be my friend, the pale milkmaid Vasilisa (VASA). She's gesturing with her left hand to indicate that the store is closed (again the Yiddish *nava*), a gesture that's intended for a figure we are familiar with by now, the wet nurse NAMA, who has turned up there wanting to go to the store.

5. NAVÁNAVÁSAMÁ: Aha, NAVA again. For a brief moment an enormous, transparent human head comes into view near the Sretenski Gates. It's swaying back and forth across the street like a pendulum (my set image for remembering the word *no*). I can see another head just like it swinging back and forth below, near the Kuznetsky Bridge, while in the center of Dzerzhinskaya Square an imposing figure suddenly comes into view—the statue of the Russian merchant woman (SAMA). *Sama,* you understand, is a term that's often used by Russian writers to describe a proprietress.

6. NAMÁSAMÁVANÁ: It would be dangerous for me to use the wet nurse and the merchant woman again, so instead I make my way down along the lane leading to the theater, where in the public garden near the Bolshoi Theater I see the seated figure of the Biblical Naomi. She stands up, and a large white samovar (SAMA) suddenly appears in her hands. She's carrying it to a tub (VANA) [Russian: *vanna*] which is on the pavement near the Orient Movie Theater. It's a tin tub, white on the inside, the outer part a greenish color.

7. SAMÁSAVÁNÁ: How simple it all becomes! I see

the massive figure of the merchant woman (*Sama*) clothed in a white shroud now (SAVANA) [Russian: *savan*, "shroud"]. She steps out of the tub and from where I'm standing I can see her back. She's heading toward the Museum of History. What will I find there? We shall see in a moment.

8. NASÁMAVÁMANÁ: What nonsense! I have to spend more time working out combinations than simply remembering. NASA—what I get turns out to be an ethereal image that doesn't work. So I grab hold of the next part of the word. Interesting, isn't it, what happens? In Hebrew *n'shama* means "soul." This is what I take for NASAMA. When I was a child the image I had of a soul was that of animal lungs and livers, which I often saw on the kitchen table. What happens, then, is that near the entrance to the museum I see a table with a "soul" lying on it—that is, lungs and liver, and also a bowl of cream of wheat. An Oriental is standing near the center of the table screaming at the soul: "Vai-vai" (VA)—"I'm sick of cream of wheat!" (MANA) [Russian: *mannaya kasha,* "cream of wheat"].

9. SANÁMAVÁNAMÁ: How naïve of them to try and provoke me like this. I recognize this right off as the scene near the Sukharevaya Tower (the scene for the third word I'd been given), only that here the particle MA has been added to the end of the word. I set up the very image I used before, except that I place it in the area between the Museum of History and the gate surrounding the Alexandrovsky Gardens. The image is of the woman nursing a baby, here a "mama" (MA). She's sitting on that slab I'd seen before.

10. VANÁSANÁVANÁ: I could go on like this forever! In the Alexandrovsky Gardens, on the main path, there

are two white porcelain tubs (that's to distinguish them from the tub I used in No. 6). These represent the syllables VANA VANA. Between them stands an attendant (SANA) [Russian: *sanitarka,* "patient"] dressed in a white uniform. And that's all there is to that one!

There is certainly no need for us to quote further from the record to demonstrate how S. replaced the monotonous alternation of syllables in this series with rich visual images that he could subsequently "read off" at will. On April 6, 1944, eight years after obtaining this record from him, I had occasion to ask S. to repeat this performance (once again without giving him prior warning). He had no difficulty whatsoever and came through with a faultless reproduction.

The excerpts I have quoted from the records on S. may give the impression that what S. accomplished was an extremely logical (if highly individualistic) reworking of the material he had to remember. But, in actual fact, nothing could be further from the truth. The enormous and truly masterful job S. did here, which the many examples quoted amply demonstrate, was essentially an operation he performed on his images, or as we have termed it in the heading of this section, a technique of eidetic images. But this is far different from using logical means to rework information received. In fact, although S. was exceptionally skilled at breaking down material into meaningful images, which he would carefully select, he proved to be quite inept at logical organization. The devices he used for his technique of eidetic images in no way resembled the logic of typical mnemonic devices (the development and psychological structure of which have been examined in numerous research studies).* All this points to a distinct type of dissociation that S. and other people with highly developed capacities for figurative memory exhibit: a tendency to rely exclusively on images and to overlook any possibility of using logical means of recall. This type of dissociation can be demonstrated quite simply in S.'s case, and we need cite only two of the experiments that were designed to examine this.

Late in the 1920's, when we first started working with S., the psychologist L. S. Vygotsky gave him a series of words to recall among which were several names of birds. In 1930, A. N. Leontiev, who was then doing some research on S.'s memory, asked him to recall a series of words that included types of liquids. When the experiments were over, S. was asked to enumerate the names of birds that had

* See A. N. Leontiev: *The Development of Memory* (Moscow, Academy Communist Education, 1931), and *Problems of Mental Development* (Moscow, Academy of Pedagogical Sciences, 1959); and A. A. Smirnov, *The Psychology of Recall* (Moscow, Academy of Pedagogical Sciences, 1948).

appeared in the first series, and the words designating liquids that had come up in the second series.

At that time S. still recalled material largely "in terms of lines," and the job of isolating those words in the series which formed one distinct category was simply beyond him. He had failed to note that among the words for recall were some that were *related in meaning,* a fact he recognized only after he had "read off" all the words in the series and had a chance to compare them.

A similar situation occurred several years later at one of S.'s performances. He was given a chart containing the following series of numbers for recall (see Table 3). With an intense effort of concentration he proceeded to recall the entire series of numbers through his customary devices of visual recall, unaware that the numbers in the series progressed in a simple logical order:

TABLE 3

| 1 | 2 | 3 | 4 |
|---|---|---|---|
| 2 | 3 | 4 | 5 |
| 3 | 4 | 5 | 6 |
| 4 | 5 | 6 | 7 |
|   |   |   | etc. |

As he later remarked:

If I had been given the letters of the alphabet arranged in a similar order, I wouldn't have noticed their arrangement. To be frank, I simply would have gone on and memorized them, although I might have become aware of it listening to the sounds of my own voice reading off the series. But I definitely wouldn't have noticed it earlier.

What better proof could one have of the discrepancy between S.'s recall and the logical ordering of material that comes so naturally to any mature mind?

We have covered practically all the information we obtained from experiments and conversations with S. about his prodigious memory, which seemed so obvious in the devices it used and yet remained so unfathomable to us. We had learned a great deal about the intricate structure of his memory: that it had formed as an accumulation of complex synesthetic impressions which he retained throughout the years; that added to its already rich figurative nature, his masterful use of eidetic images converted each sound complex into graphic images while at the same time allowing for a free flow of the old synesthetic reactions. Further, we knew that S. could remember numbers (which he regarded as the simplest type of material) through spontaneous visual recall; that he had to deal with words in terms of the images these evoked; but that when it came to remembering meaningless sounds or sound combinations, he would revert to an ex-

tremely primitive type of synesthesia—remembering these in terms of "lines" and "splashes." In
addition, he would sometimes apply his technique
of "coding the material into images," a technique
he mastered in his career as a professional
mnemonist.

Yet, how little we actually knew about his prodigious memory! How, for example, were we to explain the tenacious hold these images had on his
mind, his ability to retain them not only for years
but for decades? Similarly, what explanation was
there for the fact that the hundreds and thousands
of series he recalled did not have the effect of in-
hibiting one another, but that S. could select at
will any series ten, twelve, or even seventeen years
after he had originally memorized it? How had he
come by this capacity for indelible memory traces?

We have already pointed out that the established
ideas on memory simply did not hold for S. In his
case, traces left by one stimulus did not inhibit
those of another; they showed no sign of becoming
extinguished with time, nor did they become any
less selective with the years. It was impossible to
establish a point of limit to the capacity or the dura-
tion of his memory, or to find in him any indication
of the dynamics whereby memory traces are extinguished in the course of time. Similarly, we found
no indication of the "factor of the edge," whereby

people tend to remember the first and last elements in a series better than the elements in the middle. What is more, the phenomenon of reminiscence, a tendency for seemingly extinguished traces to come to light after a brief period of quiescence, also seemed to be lacking in S.'s case.

As noted earlier, his recall could more easily be explained in terms of factors governing *perception and attention* than in terms applicable to memory. He failed, for example, to reproduce a word if his attention had been distracted or he had been unable "to see" it clearly. His recollection hinged on factors such as the degree of lighting present, the size and positioning of an image, on whether or not an image was obscured by a blur that might turn up if someone's voice suddenly intruded on his awareness.

However, S.'s memory could not be construed as identical with the type of "eidetic memory" studied in such detail in scientific psychology thirty or forty years ago. For one thing, S. never substituted a positive for a negative afterimage in a series, a characteristic feature of "eideticism"; he also had far greater mobility with his images in that they could be made to serve his purposes. Added to this, synesthesia made his memory far more complex and distinctive than the usual type of eidetic memory.

Despite the highly intricate technique S. had developed for using eidetic images, his memory remained a striking example of spontaneous recall. Granted that he imparted certain meanings to these images which he could draw upon; he nonetheless continued to *see* the images and to experience them synesthetically. And he had no need for logical organization, for the associations *his* images produced reconstituted themselves whenever he revived the original situation in which something had been registered in his memory.

There is no question that S.'s exceptional memory was an innate characteristic, an element of his individuality, and that the techniques he used were merely superimposed on an existing structure and did not "simulate" it with devices other than those which were natural to it.*

So far, we have been describing peculiarities S. demonstrated in recalling individual elements such

---

* There is some evidence that S.'s parents demonstrated peculiarities of memory similar to those described here. According to S. when his father owned a bookstore, he could easily recall where any book was located; and his mother, a devout Jewish woman, could quote long paragraphs from the Torah. According to information we obtained in 1936 from Professor P. Dahle, who made observations of S.'s family, a nephew also had a remarkable memory. However, we do not have enough reliable information to conclude that S.'s memory was by nature genotypic.

as numbers, sounds, and words. The question remained whether these held true for his recall of more complex material—descriptions of people, events, passages in books.

S. had often complained that he had a poor memory for faces: "They're so changeable," he had said. "A person's expression depends on his mood and on the circumstances under which you happen to meet him. People's faces are constantly changing; it's the different shades of expression that confuse me and make it so hard to remember faces."

S.'s synesthetic reactions, which in the experiments described earlier had aided his recall, here became an obstacle to memory. For unlike others, who tend to single out certain features by which to remember faces (a process psychology has yet to deal with adequately), S. saw faces as changing patterns of light and shade, much the same kind of impression a person would get if he were sitting by a window watching the ebb and flow of the sea's waves.* Who, indeed, could possibly "recall" all the fluctuations of the waves' movements?

It may strike the reader as no less surprising to

* We must bear in mind that even the research on pathological cases of people who have difficulty remembering faces—the so-called agnosia for faces, or "prozopagnosia" (numerous instances of which have been written up in neurological journals)—offers no real basis for understanding this complicated process.

learn that S.'s grasp of *entire passages* in a text was far from good. We have already pointed out that, on first acquaintance, S. struck one as a disorganized and rather dull-witted person, an impression that was even more marked whenever he had to deal with a story that had been read to him. If the story was read at a fairly rapid pace, S.'s face would register confusion and finally utter bewilderment. "No," he would say. "This is too much. Each word calls up images; they collide with one another, and the result is chaos. I can't make anything out of this. And, then, there's also your voice . . . another blur . . . then everything's muddled."

S. tried reading at a slower pace, working out some order for his images, and, as we shall see from the excerpt that follows, performing a far more difficult and exhausting job on the material than others do for whom the written word does not summon up such graphic images; who operate more simply and directly by singling out key points in a passage—those that offer a maximum of information.

The following remarks are from a record of a conversation we had with S. on September 14, 1936:

Last year I was read an assignment having to do with a merchant who had sold so many meters of fabric . . .

As soon as I heard the words *merchant* and *sold,* I saw both the shop and the storekeeper, who was standing behind the counter with only the upper part of his body visible to me. He was dealing with a factory representative. Standing at the door of the shop I could see the buyer, whose back was toward me. When he moved off a little to the left, I saw not only the factory but also some account books—details that had nothing to do with the assignment. So I couldn't get the gist of the story.

And here's another example. Last year when I was chairman of a union organization I had to investigate whatever conflicts came up . . . Once they were describing some speeches that had been given in a circus tent in Tashkent, and others that were delivered at a meeting in Moscow . . . I saw all the details . . . Mentally I transported myself to Moscow and Tashkent. But this is just what I have to avoid doing. It's unnecessary. It doesn't matter whether the negotiations were held in Tashkent or elsewhere. What is important are the conditions they're describing. I was forced to block off everything that wasn't essential by covering it over in my mind with a large canvas.

## THE ART OF FORGETTING

This brings us to the last issue we had to clarify to get a fuller picture of S.'s memory. Though the problem itself is paradoxical, and the solution still difficult to understand, we will have to attempt some description at this point.

Many of us are anxious to find ways to improve our memories; none of us have to deal with the problem of how to forget. In S.'s case, however, precisely the reverse was true. The big question for him, and the most troublesome, was how he could learn to forget.

In the passages quoted above, we had our first glimpse of the problems S. ran into, trying to understand and recall a text. There were numerous details in the text, each of which gave rise to new images that led him far afield; further details produced still more details, until his mind was a virtual chaos. How could he avoid these images, prevent himself from seeing details which kept him from understanding a simple story? This was the way he formulated the problem.

Moreover, in his work as a professional mnemonist he had run into another problem. How could he learn *to forget* or *to erase* images he no longer needed? The solution to the first problem proved to be simple enough, for as S. continued to work on his technique of using images for recall, he tended to make increasingly greater use of shorthand versions of them, which automatically cut out many superfluous details. As he described it:

Here's what happened yesterday when I was listening on the radio to the account of Levanevsky's arrival.

Before, I would have seen everything: the airport, the crowds, the police cordon that had been set up . . . This doesn't happen now. I don't see the airport and it makes no difference to me whether Levanevsky landed in Tushino or in Moscow. All I see is a small segment of the Leningrad Highway, the most convenient place to meet him . . . What matters to me now is to catch every word he says; it's of no account where the event takes place. But if this had happened two years ago I would have been upset at not seeing the airport and all the other details. I'm glad now that I see only what's essential. The setup isn't important; what appears now are the necessary items, not all the minor circumstances. And this represents a great saving.

In time S.'s attempts to focus his attention, to isolate the essential details as a basis on which to generalize to the whole, brought results. Earlier, he would often have to "screen off what he had seen" by covering it with a "thick canvas," whereas at this stage he automatically screened off excess details by singling out key points of information which he used for his shorthand method of coding images.

The second problem, however, was more difficult to solve. S. frequently gave several performances an evening, sometimes in the same hall, where the charts of numbers he had to recall were written on the one blackboard there and then erased before the next performance. This led to certain problems, which he described as follows:

I'm afraid I may begin to confuse the individual performances. So in my mind I erase the blackboard and cover it, as it were, with a film that's completely opaque and impenetrable. I take this off the board and listen to it crunch as I gather it into a ball. That is, after each performance is over, I erase the board, walk away from it, and mentally gather up the film I had used to cover the board. As I go on talking to the audience, I feel myself crumpling this film into a ball in my hands. Even so, when the next performance starts and I walk over to that blackboard, the numbers I had erased are liable to turn up again. If they alternate in a way that's even vaguely like the order in one of the previous performances, I might not catch myself in time and would read off the chart of numbers that had been written there before.

(From a letter of 1939.)

How was S. to deal with this? During the early stages, his attempts to work out a technique of forgetting were of an extremely simple nature. Why, he reasoned, couldn't he use some external means to help him forget—write down what he no longer wished to remember. This may strike others as odd, but it was a natural enough conclusion for S. "People jot things down so they'll remember them," he said. "This seemed ridiculous to me, so I decided to tackle the problem my own way." As he saw it, once he had written a thing down, he would have no need to remember it; but if he were without means of writing it down, he'd commit it to memory.

Writing something down means I'll know I won't have to remember it . . . So I started doing this with small matters like phone numbers, last names, errands of one sort or another. But I got nowhere, for in my mind I continued to see what I'd written . . . Then I tried writing all the notes on identical kinds of paper, using the same pencil each time. But it still didn't work.

He went further and started to discard and then burn the slips of paper on which he had jotted down things he wished to forget. Here for the first time we have evidence of something we shall have occasion to return to later in this account: that S.'s richly figurative imagination was not sharply cut off from reality; rather, he turned to objects in the external world when he needed a means to work out some mental operation.

The "magical act of burning" he tried proved of no use to him. And after he had burned a piece of paper with some numbers he wanted to forget and discovered he could still see traces of the numbers on the charred embers, he was desperate. Not even fire could wipe out the traces he wanted to obliterate!

The problem of forgetting, which had not been solved by his naïve attempt to burn his notes, became a torment for him. Just when he thought a solution was unattainable, however, something occurred which proved effective, though it remained as unfathomable to him as it did to those of us who were studying him.

One evening—it was the 23rd of April—I was quite exhausted from having given three performances and was wondering how I'd ever get through the fourth. There before me I could see the charts of numbers appearing from the first three performances. It was a terrible problem. I thought: I'll just take a quick look and see if the first chart of numbers is still there. I was afraid somehow that it wouldn't be. I both did and didn't want it to appear . . . And then I thought: the chart of numbers isn't turning up now and it's clear why—it's because I don't want it to! Aha! That means if I don't want the chart to show up it won't. And all it took was for me to realize this!

Odd as it may seem, this brought results. It may very well be that S. had become fixated on an *absence of images,* and that had something to do with it. Possibly, too, his attention had been diverted, or the image was inhibited, and the added effect of autosuggestion was enough to destroy it. It seems pointless to conjecture about a phenomenon that has remained inexplicable. What we do have is evidence of the results it achieved.

At that moment I felt I was free. The realization that I had some guarantee against making mistakes gave me more confidence. I began to speak more freely, could even permit myself the luxury of pausing when I felt like it, for I knew that if I didn't want an image to appear, it wouldn't. I felt simply wonderful . . .

This just about exhausts our information on S.'s phenomenal memory: the role synesthesia played in it; his technique of using images on the one hand or of negating them (the mechanisms involved here still as strange and difficult to understand as ever). All of which brings us to another side of this story which we will turn to now.

We have discussed S.'s habits of perception and recall: the amazing precision of his memory; the tenacious grip that images, once evoked, had on his mind. We have also observed the peculiar structure of these images and the operations S. had to perform on them to make them serve his purposes. There remains for us to explore S.'s inner world, to get some idea of his personality and his manner of thinking.

What impact did the various facets of S.'s memory

which we have described have on his grasp of things, on the particular world he lived in? Were his habits of thought like other people's, or were there qualities in the man himself, in his behavior and personality, that were quite unique?

Here begins an account of phenomena so amazing that we will many times be left with the feeling little Alice had after she slipped through the looking glass and found herself in a strange wonderland.

# 4

## *His World*

An individual lives in a world of people and things: he sees objects, hears sounds, grasps the meaning of words. Were S.'s experiences of these like any ordinary man's, or was his a world quite different from our own?

### PEOPLE AND THINGS

S.'s extraordinary memory gave him one distinct advantage: he had recollections that dated back to infancy, memories others of us may simply never have formed or have lost because of the vast number of subsequent impressions that displaced them: possibly, too, our impressions failed to settle at such an early stage of life because our basic tool of memory, speech, had not yet developed then.

What recollections do we generally have of early childhood? Some picture, perhaps, pasted to the top of a toy chest? The steps of a staircase where we sat as a child? An impression of a quilt we had, the sense of what it felt like to be bundled in it?

It is no wonder that S.'s memories of early childhood were incomparably richer than ours. For his memory was never transformed into an apparatus for reshaping reminiscences into words, which is what happens to others of us at a fairly early age. Rather, his memory continued to summon up spontaneously images that formed part of an early period of awareness. And we can more or less trust his accounts, though we need not take everything he says on faith but can try to verify some of it. We ought, however, to follow closely the scenes he conjures up, if not the facts, which are always open to question, to note the style in which he renders them, a style that was typical of S. even at the time we knew him.

... I was very young then ... not even a year old perhaps ... What comes to mind most clearly is the furniture in the room, not all of it, I can't remember that, but the corner of the room where my mother's bed and my cradle were. A cradle is a small bed with bars on both sides, has curved wickerwork on the under part, and it rocks . . . I remember that the wallpaper in the room was brown and the bed white . . . I can see my mother taking me in her arms, then she puts me down again . . . I sense movement . . . a feeling of warmth, then an unpleasant sensation of cold.

Light is something I remember very clearly. During the day it looked like "this," afterwards, like "that"—twilight. Then came the yellow light of the lamp—it looked like "this."

(Record of August 1934.)

Thus far, S.'s memories add up to no more than the kinds of images any one of us could easily conjure up, except that for one person these might be more clear-cut, for another more diffuse. But one detects certain other notes in his story. The distinct images of childhood tend to recede into the background and what takes over are vague synesthetic sensations, a state in which there is no real borderline between perceptions and emotions; where images of the external world blend and become part of diffuse experiences; where sensations seem so vague and shifting it is hard to find words with which to convey them.

This is the sense I had of my mother: up to the time I began to recognize her, it was simply a feeling—"This is good." No form, no face, just something bending

over me, from which good would come . . . Pleasant
. . . Seeing my mother was like looking at something
through the lens of a camera. At first you can't make
anything out, just a round cloudy spot . . . then a
face appears, then its features become sharper.

My mother picks me up. I don't see her hands. All
I have is a sense that after the blur appears, something
is going to happen to me. They are picking me up. Now
I see their hands. I feel something both pleasant and
unpleasant . . . It must have been that when they
wiped me, they did it kind of roughly, and it didn't
feel good . . . or when they took me out of my crib,
particularly in the evening. I lie there and it feels like
"this" . . . Soon it will be different—like "this." I'm
scared, I cry, and the sound of my own crying only
makes me cry harder . . . Even then I understood that
after "this" feeling there would be noise, then stillness.
Right after that I could feel a pendulum, a rocking
back and forth . . .

(Record of August 1934.)

I see my mother clearly, vividly—a cloudy spot, then
something pleasant, then a face. After that, movement.
My father I recognized by his voice. Mother was on
one side of my cradle and was rocking me, while my
father rocked from the other side and blocked the light
coming from there. He must have come up to me—
that's why it grew dark. He'd come over from the side
of the room where the light was . . .

And this must have been when I had a smallpox
vaccination . . . I remember seeing a mass of fog,
then of colors. I know this means there was noise, most
likely a conversation or something like that . . . But

I don't feel any pain . . . I see myself in my mother's bed, first with my head toward the wall, then facing the door . . . I recognize the sound my own voice makes. I know that after this there'll be noise—it must be me crying . . . They are doing something to me. After the noise, a haze. Then it will feel "this way," then "that way."

This wasn't the impression I had of wetting the bed . . . I didn't know whether it was good or bad . . . I remember how the bed started to get wet. First a pleasant feeling, a feeling of warmth, then of cold, then something that doesn't feel very good, it burns. I start to cry . . . They didn't punish me . . . I remember one time—it was when I slept in the bed with my mother, but I'd already learned how to climb out. I remember Mother pointing to a spot on the bed. I can hear her voice. Most likely I could only babble then . . .

. . . And there was something else, something nasty, cold, a sensation I had of a spot, like the one you see when they sit you on the potty over there near the door close to the stove. I'm crying. It seems to me when they make me sit on the potty, I don't have to go any more. I was afraid of it . . . On the inside it's white, outside it has a greenish color, but in the middle, on the enamel part inside, there's a big black splotch . . . I think it looks like a cockroach on the wall. Then I thought it was *a zhuk.**

(Record of September 1934.)

It is difficult to say whether elements in this description go back to actual exepriences S. had in

* His association is with *zhuk* (the Russian for "beetle"). [Tr.]

childhood or whether they reflect the impressions that were peculiar to him even as an adult, at the time I knew him. Both explanations are possible, and it would be pointless to spend time deliberating, for one thing is certain: S. continued to have diffuse synesthetic reactions which, according to neurologists, hold true only for adults with the most primitive "protopathic" kind of sensitivity. What is more, these characterized almost every sensation he experienced, which is why it was so difficult in his case to locate any dividing line between one sensation and another, or between sensations and actual experiences of events. Note, for example, the following:

. . . I was ten or eleven years old and was rocking my sister to sleep. Since there were a lot of children in our family, I, being second from the oldest, often had to rock the younger ones to sleep . . . I had already sung all the songs I knew. (I had to sing in a loud voice, since it has to be foggy if one's going to fall asleep.) But why was she taking so long to fall asleep? I closed my eyes and tried to sense why it was she couldn't fall asleep. Finally I guessed the reason . . . Perhaps it was also because of *a zhuk?* So I got a towel, put it over her eyes . . . and she fell asleep.
(Record of September 1934.)

Almost all the qualities that most concern us about S.'s memory are to be found in this excerpt:

synesthetic reactions ("I had to sing in a loud voice, since it has to be foggy if one's going to fall asleep"); diffuse, childlike experiences of fear; the attempt to penetrate another person's awareness by closing one's eyes and picturing to oneself what might be troubling the other person (an aspect of S.'s behavior we will return to). And, if we are to believe S., all this went on in the mind of a ten- to eleven-year-old boy. In fact these synesthetic reactions and diffuse experiences were not confined to his boyhood; they persisted into adult life. Indeed, one can find repeated instances of them in analyzing S.'s habits of perceptions and certain characteristic features of his conscious life. The following are just a few examples of accounts he gave us.

I heard the bell ringing. A small round object rolled right before my eyes . . . my fingers sensed something rough like a rope . . . Then I experienced a taste of salt water . . . and something white.

(Record of February 1936.)

Here every sensation is aroused: the bell not only summons up a direct visual image, it also has qualities of touch, is colored white, and has a salty taste. These synesthetic elements persisted with every impression of the external world.

. . . I'm sitting in a restaurant—there's music. You know why they have music in restaurants? Because it changes the taste of everything. If you select the right kind of music, everything tastes good. Surely people who work in restaurants know this . . .

And further:

. . . I always experience sensations like these. When I ride in a trolley I can feel the clanging it makes in my teeth. So one time I went to buy some ice cream, thinking I'd sit there and eat it and not have this clanging. I walked over to the vender and asked her what kind of ice cream she had. "Fruit ice cream," she said. But she answered in such a tone that a whole pile of coals, of black cinders, came bursting out of her mouth, and I couldn't bring myself to buy any ice cream after she'd answered that way . . .

Another thing: If I read when I eat, I have a hard time understanding what I'm reading—the taste of the food drowns out the sense . . .

(Record of May 1939.)

I decide what I'm going to eat according to the name of the food, the sound of the word. It's silly to say mayonnaise tastes good. The *z* (as in the Russian spelling) ruins the taste—it's not an appealing sound . . . For a long time I couldn't eat hazel grouse. A grouse is a hopping thing. And if a menu is badly written, I simply can't eat—the menu seems so filthy . . .

Here's what happened one time. I went into a place to eat and the waiter asked if I'd like some biscuits. But then he brought me rolls . . . "No," I thought, "these aren't biscuits"; the *r* and *zh* sounds in biscuits

[Russian: *korzhiki*] are such hard, crunching, biting sounds . . ."

(Record of May 1939.)

These experiences did not apply to S.'s entire world, but here there definitely is no dividing line between color and sound, between sensations of taste and of touch. Rather, he senses smooth, cold sounds and rough colors; salty shades and bright, clear, or biting smells, all so intertwined and fused that it is hard to distinguish one sensation from the other.

This brings us to another topic. What effect had synesthesia on S.'s perception of speech? What did words mean to him? Were there in words, too, those same admixtures of synesthesia which converted noise into "puffs of steam" and altered the taste of a dish if it were mentioned in an "unpleasant" or "biting" tone of voice? What did S. make of the meaning of words?

WORDS

We have already seen how S. interpreted meaning several pages back with his reference to *a zhuk,* an expression he had used in childhood. What did this word, which when he first used it meant "beetle" but which later took on such a broad range of meaning, actually denote for him?

. . . *A zhuk*—that's a dented piece in the potty . . .
It's a piece of rye bread . . . And in the evening
when you turn on the light, that's also *a zhuk,* for the
entire room isn't lit up, just a small area, while everything else remains dark—*a zhuk.* Warts are also *a zhuk*
. . . Now I see them sitting me before a mirror.
There's noise, laughter. There are my eyes staring at
me from the mirror—dark—they're also *a zhuk* . . .
Now I'm lying in my crib . . . I hear a shout, noise,
threats. Then someone's boiling something in the
enamel teakettle. It's my grandmother making coffee.
First she drops something red into the kettle, then
takes it out—*a zhuk.* A piece of coal—that's also *a
zhuk* . . . I see them lighting candles on the Sabbath.
A candle is burning in the holder, but some of the
tallow hasn't melted yet. The wick flickers and goes
out. Then everything turns black. I'm scared, I cry—
this is also *a zhuk* . . . And when people are sloppy
pouring tea, and the drops miss the pot and land on
the plates, that's also *a zhuk.*

(Record of September 1934.)

What a familiar ring all this has for psychologists. Shtumpf observed that his small son used
*kwa* to mean a duck, an eagle engraved on a coin,
and the coin itself. Or take the expression we are
all familiar with, the *khe* sound a child uses to
designate not only a cat and its fur but also a sharp
stone he has scratched himself on. There is definitely an authentic ring of childhood in S.'s stories.
Yet whereas the broad range of meaning children

attach to words is a common enough phenomenon, one quickly detects new notes in these familiar motifs as S. presents them.*

. . . Take the word *mama,* or *ma-me,* as we used to say when I was a child. It's a bright haze. *Ma-me* and all women—they're something bright . . . So is milk in a glass, and a white milk jug, and a white cup. They're all like a white cloud.

But, then, take the word *gis* [Yiddish: "pour"]. That came up later. What it meant to me was a sleeve, something trailing down, long, the stream that flows when people are pouring tea . . . And the reflection of a face in the polished surface of the samovar—that's also *gis.* It glistens like the sound *s* . . . But an oval face is like a stream of water, like a hand in a sleeve slowly lowering to pour tea...

(Record of September 1934.)

What we find here is not simply that words have a wide range of meaning. We are well aware that a word means something, that it designates a sign which is extended to cover a range of things—whatever evidences this sign. But a word is also expressed through a complex of sounds which may vary with the voice of the speaker. For S., both the sound of a word and the voice of the speaker had a distinct color and taste that produced "puffs

* A. R. Luria and F. Y. Yudovich, *Speech and the Development of Higher Psychological Functions in the Child* (London, Stagler Press, 1959).

of steam," "splashes," and "blurs." Some sounds appeared to him as smooth and white; others as orange and sharp as arrows. Consequently, for him the meaning of words was also reflected in the sounds they embodied. This is quite a different form of extended reference, based on the synesthetic sense one has of a word, of its sound qualities.

People generally do not pay much attention to the phonetic elements of words, which tend to fade into the background for them; for they are primarily concerned with meaning and usage. Hence we are not likely to get a sense either of harmony or of contradiction by terming one tree a "pine," another a "fir," a third a "birch."

S.'s experiences, on the other hand, were quite different. He distinctly felt that the sound and sense of certain words corresponded exactly; that there were other words which needed some revising; and still other words whose meaning struck him as totally unnatural, words he thought must surely have come into the language through some misunderstanding. Note, for example, the following descriptions.

. . . I was ill with scarlatina . . . I had come back from Hebrew school with a headache and my mother had said: "He has *heets* [Yiddish: "fever"]. True enough! *Heets* is intense, like lightning . . . and I had

such a sharp orange light coming out of my head. So
that word's right for sure!

. . . But take the word *holz* [Yiddish: "firewood"].
It just doesn't fit. *Holz* has such a brilliant hue, a ray
of light around it . . . Yet it's supposed to mean "log"
. . . No, that's wrong—some misunderstanding.

. . . Then there's the word "pig" [Russian: *svinya*].
Now, I ask you, can this really be a pig? *Svi-n-ya*—
it's so fine, so elegant . . . But what a difference when
you come to *khavronya* [Russian: "sow"] or *khazzer*
[Yiddish: "pig"]. That's really it—the *kh* sound makes
me think of a fat greasy belly, a rough coat caked
with dried mud, a *khazzer!* . . .*

. . . And when I was five they took me to the Hebrew school to begin studying. Before that, the teacher
had been to our apartment. So when my parents told
me: "You'll go to school and study with Kamerazh,"
I figured this meant the man I'd seen, the one with
the dark beard who was dressed in a long coat and
broad-brimmed hat. Clearly this was Kamerazh, except
that the word *rebe* [Yiddish: "teacher"] just didn't fit
him . . . *Rebe* is something white, whereas he was so
dark.

. . . And then there's the word *Nebuchadnezzar* [Yid-
dish pronunciation: Nabukhadneitser] . . . No, this is
some mistake. He was so wicked, he could tear a lion
to pieces. If it were *Nebukhadreitser,* that would really
suit him!

. . . As for *shnits* [Yiddish: "pointed"], that's all
right. It had to be something thin and sharp.

* The term in Yiddish meaning the animal itself and, more exten-
sively, anything foul or gluttonous. Hence a more emotive word
than either the English or the Russian. [Tr.]

. . . And *dog* [Russian: "great Dane"] is also un-
derstandable . . . It's big and should have that sort of
word . . .

. . . But take the word *samovar*. Of course it's just
sheer luster—not from the samovar, but from the letter
*s*. But the Germans use the word *Teemaschine*. That's
not right. *Tee* is a falling sound—it's here! Oi! I was
afraid of that, it's on the floor . . . So how could
*Teemaschine* mean the same thing as *samovar?* . . .

(Records of September and October 1934.)

For S., the meaning of a word had somehow to
fit its sound. Otherwise, he could easily be thrown
off balance.

Our family doctor was a man by the name of Dr.
Tigger. *"Me darf rufen den Tigger,"* my parents would
say. I thought some tall cane would surely come walking in, because the *e* and *r* sounds drop downward. But
who was he? "The doctor," they said. Yet when I saw
the word *doctor,* it looked like a round honey cake
with bunches of some sort hanging down, and I put
this on top of the cane. When a tall, ruddy-looking
fellow arrived, I looked him over and thought to myself: "No, he's not the one" . . .

(Record of March 31, 1938.)

And here is a description of a similar instance of a
disparity S. found, except that this came up when
he was much older.

. . . I was going to school then . . . We were reading about Afanasy Ivanovich and Pul'kheriya Ivanovna* having eaten biscuits with lard. I understood this had to do with food, except that a *korzhik* [Russian: "biscuit"] definitely has to be a fancy, oblong-shaped bread with twists, a *kalatch*. But once in 1931 when I was in a coffeehouse in Baku I ordered biscuits with lard. If they're biscuits, they'd have looked exactly as I've described them—no different. But the waiter served me coffee and two cookies. I told him I'd asked for biscuits, but all he said was: "That's what I gave you—biscuits with lard!" Yet it was clear these weren't biscuits; they didn't fit at all . . .

(Record of October 1934.)

The meaning of a word simply had to add up to what its sound suggested to him.

. . . For some reason the word *mutter* produces an image of a dark brown sack with folds, hanging in a vertical position. That's what I saw when I first heard the word . . . The vowel sound is the base; the consonants make up the general background setting of the word. I see the bend in the word, but the *t* and *r* sounds are dominant . . .

. . . *Milch,* though [Yiddish: "milk"], is a thin thread with a little bag attached. *Leffel* [Yiddish: "spoon"] is braided like a *hallah,* while *hallah* itself is such a hard word, you have to snap it off . . . As for *maim*

* From a Nikolai Gogol tale. [Tr.]

[Yiddish: "water"], it's a cloud . . . That *m*—it seems to drift off somewhere.

(Record of October 1934.)

S. had considerable difficulty adapting the meaning of a word to its sound, and his childlike synesthesia persisted for some time.

The sound of a word has one distinct form and color, the meaning another form and a particular weight as well, it sounds different . . . For me to come up with the right word at the right time, I have to fit all this together. On the one hand it makes for complications, but on the other, it is a way of remembering words. If I keep in mind this peculiarity of mine, that I have to adapt to the way others think, that's one thing. But if I forget this, I'm liable to give people the impression I'm a dull, senseless fellow . . .

(Record of October 1934.)

There is another aspect to interpreting words synesthetically (determining meaning, that is, through both sound and sense). Whereas certain words seem not to fit the meaning they conventionally have, and therefore leave one nonplussed, the sound qualities of other words take on particular expressive force. S.'s experience of words was actually a measure of their expressiveness. No wonder, then, that S. M. Eisenstein, the producer, to whom the dynamics of expression were of such crucial importance in his own work, was so intrigued with S.

Here is an example of S.'s reaction to the tone qualities of words:

. . . I once heard that a boy had broken into a shop in Baikal and stolen a 50-kopeck piece from the cashbox. I didn't know at the time what a 50-kopeck piece [Russian: *poltinnik*] was. It seemed to me some sort of oblong-shaped object, quiet and mysterious, for after all the *p* and *t* are such dark sounds. The storekeeper gave the boy a *potch* [Yiddish: "slap"]. I knew what that was—it's not a nice word . . . But there's also *frask* [another Yiddish word for "slap"]. This sounds somewhat hollow, whereas *khlyask* [also Yiddish for "slap"] has a rather crackling sound.

(Record of May 1936.)

Perhaps the most revealing instance of the expressive power sounds had for S. was an experiment in which he tried to define for us the differences he sensed in variations of a name—a name such as Mariya, with its Russian variants: Masha, Marusya, Mary.

. . . Even now, as an adult, I interpret them all differently. Mariya, Masha, Mary—no, this is not the same woman. Manya [another variant] fits her, but not Marusya or Mary. It was a long time before I could grasp the idea that these names could all apply to the same woman. And even now I can't quite reconcile myself to it . . . Mariya has a strong build and fair skin—except for a slight flush in her cheeks. She's blond, her gestures are composed, and she has a look in her eyes that says she's up to no good. Marya is the same type, only plump, with ruddy cheeks and a big bosom . . . Masha is a bit younger, frail, wears a pink dress . . . Manya is a young woman, shapely perhaps. She's a brunette with sharp facial features and a matted complexion—no shine either on her nose or on her cheeks. So I can't understand how this could possibly be Aunt Manya . . .

I asked S. why Manya struck him as a young woman.

*N* is a nasal sound, so I don't know. But she's young. As for Musya [another variant of Mariya], that's something else again. What impresses me most is her magnificent hairdo. She's also short and shapely—probably because of the *u* sound. As for Mary, that's a very dry name . . . suggests a dark figure sitting by the window at twilight . . . So, when someone says, "Did you see Masha?" I can't get the idea right off that this can mean Masha, Manya, or Marusya. They're not the same woman . . . Sometimes it's very difficult for me to get used to the idea that a person even has such a name. At other times, well, of course it's Masha . . . of course it's her.

(Record of May 1938.)

Poets, as we know, are extremely sensitive to the expressive quality of sounds, And I remember, too,

that S. M. Eisenstein, in testing students to select
those he would train as film directors, asked them
to describe their impressions of the variations on the
name Mariya (Mariya, Mary, Marusya). He
found this an infallible way to single out those who
were keenly sensitive to the expressive force of
words.

This ability was developed to such a degree in
S. that he never failed to detect the expressive qualities of sounds. It was only natural, then, that words
which others accept as synonyms would have different meanings for him.

. . . Take the words *thief* and *rogue* [Russian: *vor* and
*zhulik*]. A thief is a very pale fellow with sunken
cheeks, a tortured expression on his face. He goes
about without a cap and his hair looks like straw. He's
poorly dressed, his pockets all ripped. All this has to
do with that *o* sound, that long *o* [pronounced *vo-or*
in Russian]. It's such a gray word. And since the Jews
don't pronounce the *r,* you get *vookh*—completely
gray. As for *rogue* [Russian: *zhulik*], that's something
else . . . This is a fellow with full shiny cheeks; he's
got a scar over one eye and a lewd look in his eyes.
When I was little, I pronounced it *zulik*. Then he
seemed to me small, sturdy, and sinewy, and the *zz*
sound was like the noise a fly makes. I thought it was
a fly buzzing on the windowpane. Later, when I realized how the word was actually pronounced, the little
fellow I'd seen grew taller.

Then there's *ganef* [Yiddish: "thief"]. He turns up

in the evening when it's growing dark and you still
haven't lit the lamp. You hear rustling—then he steals
a piece of bread from the shelf . . . That's what I
heard when I was little—some bread had been stolen
from the shelf. From where? From our pantry, most
likely . . .

. . . I could feel pity for a thief [*vor*], but a *ganef*—
never! And I could be merciful toward a *zulik*, but as
for a *zhulik*—what, that ugly mug? For other people
it depends upon how the fellow's dressed; for me it's a
question of how his face strikes me . . .

. . . Then take the words *khvorat* and *bolet* [both
mean "to be ill," in Russian]—they're different. *Bolet*
is a mild illness, whereas *khvorat* is serious. *Khvoroba*
[Russian: "ailment"] is a gray word, it drops, closes
down on a person . . . But it's possible to say of
someone that he was seriously ill and use *bolet* because
*bolezn* [noun from same root, meaning "illness"] is a
kind of haze that might issue from the person himself
and engulf him . . . But if it's said *on khvorat,* it means
the person is lying downstairs somewhere; *khvorat* is
worse than *bolet*. And if you say *on prikhvaryvayet*
[Russian: "he is unwell"], it means he's walking about
and limping . . . But this isn't related to the general
sound pattern. These are quite different things . . .

(Record of March 1938.)

With this we come on a new area of response
we have yet to explore, one that transcends the
mere "physiognomy of words."

# 5

## *His Mind*

We have examined the nature of S.'s memory and have had a brief glimpse of his inner world, enough to see that it differed in many respects from our own, being made up of striking images and composite kinds of experience. In that these experiences consisted of a variety of sensations that would fuse imperceptibly one with the other, they are difficult to render in words. We have also noted how S. organized and interpreted words, the kinds of operations he had to perform on them in order to get beyond his impressions to the actual meaning of the words.

But what kind of mind did he have? How did

he proceed to learn, to acquire knowledge and master complex intellectual operations? What distinguished his manner of thinking from other people's?

Here once again we find ourselves in a world of contradictions where, as we shall see, the advantages S. derived from his graphic, figurative manner of thinking were bound up with distinct limitations; where a wealth of thought and imagination were curiously combined with limitations of intellect.

## HIS STRONG POINTS

S. characterized his own manner of thinking as "speculative," though in fact it bore no resemblance to the abstract, speculative reasoning of rationalist philosophy. His was a mind which operated through vision—and in this sense only could it be termed "speculative."* For S. could actually see what other people think or only dimly imagine to themselves; vivid images would appear to him that were so palpable as to verge on being real. What thinking

* The Russian for "speculative" is *umozritelny*—literally, "seen with the mind." Hence the reference to it as a possible description of S.'s manner of thought. His use of the word, however unidiomatic, is curiously apt as a description of the way he operated, almost a pun on the conventional meaning of "speculative." [Tr.]

he did amounted merely to operations he would then perform on his images.

There are, of course, a number of advantages to be derived from such graphic vision (and also substantial limitations, which we will return to later). For one thing S. could become more deeply involved in a narrative, never missing a single detail and at times spotting contradictions the writers themselves had failed to notice. The following, for example, are points he picked up in some of Chekhov's stories:

. . . Here's an example of the kinds of contradictions I often find. We've all read Chekhov's story "The Malefactor." But don't you think there's something wrong at one point in the story? Just listen. The inspector says to the peasant: "Aha, I suppose you didn't know the nuts are used to fasten the rails to the ties?" Is that right? No! Yet that's what Chekhov wrote. But, you know, I can see it, see it's wrong. So I reread it. No, a "nut" simply won't do here . . .

. . . And who hasn't read "The Chameleon"? Chekhov writes: "Ochumelov came out in his new greatcoat." Later, however, we read: "When he caught sight of what was going on there, he said: 'Officer, here! Help me off with my coat!' "*. . . I thought I was mistaken and turned back to the beginning of the story, but there was the word *greatcoat* . . . So it was Chekhov who was wrong, not I . . .

* He is referring to two words for coat: *shinel,* greatcoat; and *pal'to,* simply an overcoat. [Tr.]

. . . And here's another example. Take Chekhov's story "Fat and Thin." Early in the story the gymnasium students had been wearing uniforms, for Chekhov had written: "In the beginning he hadn't worn his cap with any dash!" Later in the story, he writes: "Upon hearing the man was a general, he adjusted his cap."* You can find many instances of this sort of thing both in Chekhov's and in Sholokhov's writing. They didn't see these, but I do . . .

(Record of March 1951.)

S.'s graphic reading of stories gave him a certain perspective which the authors of say, "The Malefactor" and *The Quiet Don* lacked. Whereas the writers were concerned with ideas and the development of plot, S. could actually *see* all the details and thus would not fail to pick up any contradictions in the stories. He did not need to develop his power of observation, since it was integral to his particular kind of mind.

His graphic vision not only had the effect of making him observant; it also allowed him to solve, with an ease that was truly enviable, certain practical problems that others would have to reason through at length. These he solved quite simply, by means of his inner vision.

At one point in S.'s life, he was hired as an

* Here it is two different words for cap: *shapka,* cap; and *furazhka,* cap with a visor. [Tr.]

efficiency expert. From the following, one can see how readily he turned up solutions.

All the things I devised came to me so easily! I didn't have to rack my brains, for I could see before me what had to be done . . . Once when I arrived at a sewing factory I saw them loading bales of material in the yard. The bales were bound with selvage. In my mind I could see the workers tying these bales: they turn them over several times and then the selvage rips. I could hear the crackling sound it made as it ripped. I looked further into this and what came to mind was a rubber band, the kind one uses to tie around a notebook. That would work here, except that it would have to be a large band . . . In my mind I enlarged it until what I saw was a rubber inner tube from an automobile tire. If one were to cut this, it would be just right here. I could see this in my mind and so I suggested it to the people at the factory . . .

 . . . And here's another example. You remember when we used to have little cards with money coupons —squares with numbers indicating the values: rubles, kopecks . . . My job was to think up an easier way for people to clip out these coupons without ripping out so many others. I had an image of a man standing near the cash register. He's a wise guy. He wants to do this on the sly, not have anyone see him tearing them out . . . I spy on him. No, not that way! This way's better! And that's how I found a better solution. Problems which other people have to figure out on paper, I can do "speculatively". . .

(Record of October 1937.)

Admittedly, many of S.'s proposals were not too practical (practicality was not one of his strong points). Where, after all, could one find enough inner tubes to cut into rubber rings to use to package bales? Still, the fact that he could solve problems "speculatively" which others had to "figure out on paper" was a considerable advantage. This was particularly so in problems other people have difficulty with because their use of verbal "calculations" cuts off the possibility of visualizing a solution. The following illustrates S.'s manner of proceeding.

You remember the mathematical joke: There were two books on a shelf, each 400 pages long. A bookworm gnawed through from the first page of the first volume to the last page of the second. How many pages did he gnaw through? You would no doubt say 800—400 pages of the first volume and 400 of the second. But I see the answer right off! He only gnaws through the two bindings. What I see is this: the two books are standing on the shelf, the first on the left, the second to the right of it. The worm begins at the first page and keeps going to the right. But all he finds there is the binding of the first volume and that of the second. So, you see, he hasn't gnawed through anything except the two bindings . . .

(Record of May 1934.)

The mechanisms by which graphic thinking operates can be seen even more clearly in S.'s treatment of problems in which certain abstract ideas that constitute the given are in conflict with any attempt to visualize a solution. Since S. never dealt in abstractions, he was spared this conflict, and solutions that prove difficult for others came to him quite easily.

. . . It was at Bronnaya Street, where we had a small room, that I met the mathematician G. He told me how he solved problems and suggested I try one. He was sitting there in the room, and I was standing, when he began. "Imagine," he said, "that there's an apple in front of you and you have to tie it tightly all around with a string or a thong. What you should end up with by way of an answer is a circumference having a certain length. Now I'll add one meter to the length of that circumference. The new circumference will be equal to that of the apple plus one meter. Take hold of the apple again; it's clear that there's quite a distance between it and the string."

As he was telling me this, I could see the apple in my mind, see myself bending over and tying it tightly around with the string. When he mentioned the word *thong,* I saw that, too. And when he talked about an additional meter, I had an image of a piece of thong . . . no, that's not true . . . a whole thong, which I made a circle out of and in the middle of it I placed the apple.

Then he said: "Picture to yourself the earth's globe." At first I saw a large terrestrial globe—hills, mountains—all encircled with the thong. "Now," he said, "let us add one meter to the thong. You should get a certain distance between it and the globe. What will this amount to?" What first appeared to me was this huge globe of the earth. I grabbed and tried to get hold of it, but it was too close . . . I pushed it farther away and then transformed it into a small globe without a pedestal. But this didn't work either, for it resembled the apple I had seen before. Then suddenly the room we were in disappeared and I caught sight of an enormous globe far off in the distance—several kilometers away from where I stood. Then I substituted a steel hoop for the thong (which wasn't an easy job since I had to make it fit tightly around the globe). I added a meter and saw how the hoop sprang back, leaving a space between it and the globe. But how much space was there? I had to figure this out, to convert the distance into dimensions people conventionally use. Then I saw a box near the door. I made a sphere out of it and bound it with the thong . . . Then I added exactly one meter to the corners of the box, measured exactly and cut the meter into four parts, each 25 centimeters long. For each thong, then, I would get an excess amount—the length of each side of the box plus a fourth . . . So, whatever the dimensions of the box— if each side, say, were 100 kilometers, I'd still add 25 centimeters to it. The result, then, is the four sides and an additional 25 centimeters for each. I drew the strap back along the side and came out with a measurement of 12.5 centimeters for each side. Everywhere along the box the strap was 12.5 centimeters wide of the box. Even if the box were enormous, and each side were a million centimeters long, it wouldn't make any difference. If I added one meter, there would be an additional 25 centimeters on each side . . . I then converted the box back to its normal shape. All I'd have to do was cut off the corners to convert it into a sphere, and I'd get the same result again. That's how I solved this problem.

(Record of March 1937.)

The reader, it is hoped, will forgive me for quoting at such length from the record. My one justification is that it indicates the methods S. used and shows how these enabled him to solve problems through means so different from those a person would use if he were "figuring it out on paper."

We spent hours with S. analyzing the advantages to be had from the method he used to solve arithmetical problems. His analysis of the part graphic images played in this proved enlightening. No doubt people will always have reason to rely on written computations or mental calculations to solve arithmetical problems; yet how often we are misled because we rely excusively on calculations not based on any image of the problem. Either we end up with the wrong answer or we substitute involved, uneconomical methods for one that would be quite simple. For example, we are all familiar with the difficulties we can run into with a simple problem such as: What is the weight of a brick which weighs 1 kilogram plus the weight of a half brick? Operating strictly with numbers, we could easily be misled into thinking the answer was 1.5 kilograms. This readiness to slip into formal responses was foreign to S.—indeed, impossible for him. His "inner vision," which forced him to deal with concrete *objects,* to associate numbers with graphic images, did not permit of formal solutions. Consequently, problems that create conflicts for other people were quite simple for him; he did not have to choose between formal and specific means. Here are a few illustrations of the way he handled problems.

. . . I was given the following problem to solve. A bound book costs 1 ruble, 50 kopecks. The book alone is a ruble more than the binding. What is the cost of each? I solved this quite simply. I have a book in a red binding. The price of the book alone is 1 ruble more than that of the binding. I pull out part of the book and think to myself that this costs 1 ruble. What remains is the part of the book that equals the cost of the binding—50 kopecks. Then I put this part of the book back with the other, and I get as an answer 1 ruble, 25 kopecks.

Or take another example. An engineer friend of mine gave me this problem to solve: The ages of a father and his son together add up to 47. How old were they three years ago? I see the father holding his son by the hand. They add up to 47 years. Along with them I see still another son and another father. I knock three years off for each . . . Then I think: this has to be doubled. So I multiply by 2, which gives me 6, and subtract 6 from 47.

(Record of March 1937.)

His graphic images of objects kept him from falling into the sort of errors other people can make who use formal methods to solve problems. S. was never tempted to substitute formal, numerical calculations for his original solutions. Given the following problem, he proceeded to deal with it graphically. This is the problem: The price of a notebook is four times that of a pencil. The pencil is 30 kopecks cheaper than the notebook. How much is each? S. solved the problem this way:

A notebook appears on the table with four pencils beside it:

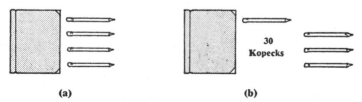

(a)                    (b)

The pencil is 30 kopecks cheaper than the notebook . . . Since three of the pencils are superfluous, they're pushed aside to the right, making room for the notebook, their equivalent value in money. Immediately after these images I see the numbers 10 and 40—the answer to the question how much the notebook and the pencil cost separately.

(From S.'s notes.)

It can readily be seen why S. could operate so quickly and simply by means of his "inner vision," whereas the use of verbal-logical means would entail supplementary abstract calculations. The devices S. used were even more apparent in his treatment of more complex problems. Let us consider two of these.

S. was given the following problem to solve: A wise man and a traveler were sitting on the grass. The traveler had 2 loaves of bread; the wise man, 3. A passer-by approached and they invited him to dine with them, dividing the bread they had into 3 equal parts. When he finished eating, the passer-by gave them 10 eggs in return for their hospitality. How did the wise man and the traveler divide the 10 eggs they received?

. . . What appeared to me were images of the two (A and B) sitting on the grass. They are joined by the passer-by (C). The three assume the form of a triangle, and in the space between them I see the loaves of bread. The people disappear and are replaced by the letters $\begin{smallmatrix} A & B \\ & C \end{smallmatrix}$ and the irregular shape of the loaves on elongated planks. The planks belonging to A are gray; B's are white. With two horizontal lines

I cut the planks into three equal groups of cubes and get the following picture:

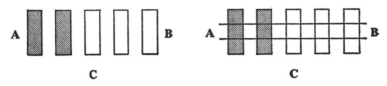

C gave them 10 eggs for the 5 cubes he had eaten. A had 6 cubes, of which he himself ate the first vertical row and 2 of the cubes in the second row. B's loaves added up to the same configuration, and he ate an equal amount. The drawing shows the number of cubes C got from each:

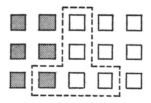

You could solve this another way. For the sake of convenience, I'll substitute rubles for eggs. The part of the bread eaten by the passer-by amounted to 10 rubles' worth. All three have eaten the same amount; therefore, the amount of bread consumed by the group adds up to 30 rubles ($10 \times 3 = 30$), whereas one loaf amounts to 6 rubles' worth ($30 \div 5 = 6$). The two loaves belonging to the traveler would amount to 12 rubles' worth ($2 \times 6 = 12$). The quantity of bread the traveler himself ate amounted to 10 rubles' worth, which means that he could have given only 2 rubles'

worth to the passer-by ($12 - 10 = 2$). The wise man had 3 loaves, or 18 rubles' worth; of these he offered the passer-by an amount equal to 8 rubles . . . A figurative solution proceeds very quickly, almost involuntarily. On the other hand, an abstract, verbal solution requires careful analysis, logical deduction, and a certain degree of intuition. But the result is the same . . .

(From S.'s notes.)

S. turned up a similar solution in response to the following problem: A man and his wife are picking mushrooms. The husband says to the wife: "Give me 7 of your mushrooms and I'll have twice as many as you!" To which the wife replies: "No, give me 7 of yours and we'll have the same amount." How many mushrooms does each have?

I could see the path in the woods. The husband tall and wearing glasses. Crooked over his elbow is a white wicker basket with mushrooms. He's grown tired . . . Aha! I conclude then that he must have picked a lot of mushrooms. His wife is standing with her back toward me (after all, he was the one who first began to speak, not she). I see myself and I see them. And it is this I, the one who is standing on the edge of the woods, who determines how many mushrooms they've picked, while the factual I, a man, not an image, spy on him to see how he figures it out.

This, then, is the first estimate. I don't know whether he has a lot of mushrooms, but I think he must, for he used the expression "twice as much." I still don't know what the situation is. But when he replies "Aha," at once it's clear to me. For when he said, "Give me 7 mushrooms," I saw a small pile of mushrooms he was putting in his basket. When she answered, he pulled these out of his basket, and I saw that the level in both baskets was the same . . .

The actual grouping of the 7 has features that are typical of 7. The fellow I saw moves off a bit and I follow him. And at once the number 14 appears. I have already determined that he was counting 14 mushrooms, for the two of us are operating in different ways: I'm working with numbers, while he converts everything into a weight, a form, an image . . .

But it isn't enough simply to take 7 mushrooms away from the husband (the bottom of his basket had slipped open and a pile of 7 mushrooms had dropped out). These have to be slipped into his wife's basket. Otherwise, he'll have 7 more than she . . . This means that altogether he has 14 more and they're in two piles. I take a quick look at what's in her basket and see that the level decreases accordingly; but when the two piles of mushrooms are added, it increases.

This is how I get a value for the first part of the problem, which had no meaning before (the statement, that is, "Give me 7 mushrooms and I'll have twice as many as you"). Their situation is as it was before: he has the two piles of mushrooms ready, but if she takes one of hers out he won't have twice as many. It won't do just to have one pile slip out of her basket—this has to be gotten into his. That means it has to be reduced by one pile if he is to have 21 more than she. When this is added to his, he'll have 28 more. And when he has 28 more, he'll then have twice as many as she! By now I can see the bottom of his basket: he has 8 piles, she has 4 . . .

At this point I start to check it through. After all, I have to translate all this into the kinds of terms people understand. All of it disappears—that is, the people leave. What appears are two black posts encircled with fog at the top (for I don't really know how many mushrooms they have). I reason it through and determine that he has more mushrooms than she. The tip of the first post pushes up higher—he has more!

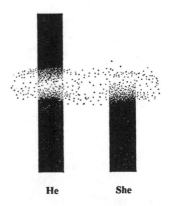

**He**        **She**

Here I'm reasoning in two ways—with numbers and with a diagram. I start to level off the two posts: I cut 7 off one post. But even when this piece has fallen off, the post is still higher. They'll be equal only when I transfer that piece to the right side. Clearly this means 14! I set the two posts up as they were before. The last piece at the top represents 14. But she says to him: "Give me 7 mushrooms and I'll be twice as tall as you!"

So I cut off another 7 from the post on the right, and he has 21 more. But I still need to add to his, so he'll have 28 more . . . Now I see that her lower piece is equal to his upper one— altogether 56. So I substract and get these figures:

$$56 - 7 = 49$$
$$28 + 7 = 35$$

(Record of January 1947.)

We have purposely given so much space to this long account of S.'s reasoning processes because it allows us to see something of his world and of the graphic "speculative" means he used to solve problems. Can there be any doubt that this was quite different from the way others would "figure it out on paper," that this was clearly a very particular realm of "speculative" thought.*

### HIS WEAK POINTS

We have glimpsed the high points of S.'s thinking. What remains is for us to explore its low points. Here the going will prove more difficult, the ways of his mind leading us through unsteady ground where at any moment we might founder.

* We will not complicate this account by citing further examples that would illustrate the advantages to be derived from graphic thinking. We have available numerous examples of problem-solving which S. described for us. Very likely these will be published elsewhere.

We have seen that S.'s graphic thinking provided a powerful base on which to operate, allowing him to carry out in his mind manipulations which others could perform only with objects. Were there not certain risks, however, in relying exclusively on figurative, particularly on synesthetic, thinking? Didn't this create obstacles with respect to certain basic cognitive functions? Let us consider these questions here.

When S. read a passage from a text, each word produced an image. As he put it: "Other people *think* as they read, but I *see* it all." As soon as he began a phrase, images would appear; as he read further, still more images were evoked, and so on.

As we mentioned earlier, if a passage were read to him quickly, one image would collide with another in his mind; images would begin to crowd in upon one another and would become contorted. How then was he to understand anything in this chaos of images? If a text were read slowly, this, too, presented problems for him. Note the difficulties he experienced:

... I was read this phrase: "N. was leaning up against a tree . . ." I saw a slim young man dressed in a dark blue suit (N., you know, is so elegant). He was standing near a big linden tree with grass and woods all around . . . But then the sentence went on: "and was peering into a shop window." Now how do you like

that! It means the scene isn't set in the woods, or in a garden, but he's standing on the street. And I have to start the whole sentence over from the beginning . . .
(Record of March 1937.)

Thus, trying to understand a passage, to grasp the information it contains (which other people accomplish by singling out what is most important), became a tortuous procedure for S., a struggle against images that kept rising to the surface in his mind. Images, then, proved an obstacle as well as an aid to learning in that they prevented S. from concentrating on what was essential. Moreover, since these images tended to jam together, producing still more images, he was carried so far adrift that he was forced to go back and rethink the entire passage. Consequently a simple passage—a phrase, for that matter—would turn out to be a Sisyphean task. These vivid, palpable images were not always helpful to S. in understanding a passage; they could just as easily lead him astray.

And this was only the beginning of the problems S. encountered in reading. As he described it:

. . . It's particularly hard if there are some details in a passage I happen to have read elsewhere. I find then that I start in one place and end up in another—everything gets muddled. Take the time I was reading *The Old World Landowners*. Afanasy Ivanovich went out on the porch . . . Well, of course, it's such a high porch, has such creaking benches . . . But, you know, I'd already come across that same porch before! It's Korobochka's porch, where Chichikov drove up! What's liable to happen with my images is that Afanasy Ivanovich could easily run into Chichikov and Korobochka! . . .*

. . . Or take another example. This one has to do with Chichikov's arrival at the hotel. I see the place, a one-story house. You enter and there's the foyer, downstairs a large reception room with a window near the doorway, to the right a table, and in the center of the room a big Russian stove . . . But I've seen this before. The fat Ivan Nikiforovich lives in this very house, and the thin Ivan Ivanovich is here too—in the garden out in front, with the filthy Gapka running about beside him. And so I've ended up with different people from the characters in the novel.

(Record of March 1937.)

Thinking in terms of images was fraught with even greater dangers. Inasmuch as S.'s images were particularly vivid and stable, and recurred thousands of times, they soon became the dominant element in his awareness, uncontrollably coming to the surface whenever he touched upon something that was linked to them even in the most general way.

* The characters he describes are from Gogol's *Dead Souls* and some of the stories in his Ukrainian tales. S.'s reading leads to a state of confusion in which characters from the different works come together in a single image. [Tr.]

These were images of his childhood: of the little house he had lived in in Rezhitsa; of the yard at Chaim Petukh's, where he could see the horses standing in the shed, where everything smelled of oats and manure. This explains why, once he had begun to read or had started one of his mental walks connected with recall, he would suddenly discover that although he had started out at Mayakovsky Square he invariably ended up at Chaim Petukh's house or in one of the public squares in Rezhitsa.

Say I began in Warsaw—I end up in Torzhok in Alter-mann's house . . . Or I'm reading the Bible. There's a passage in which Saul appears at the house of a certain sorceress. When I started reading this, the witch described in "The Night Before Christmas" appeared to me. And when I read further, I saw the little house in which the story takes place—that is, the image I had of it when I was seven years old: the bagel shop and the storage room in the cellar right next to it . . . Yet it was the Bible I had started to read . . .

(Record of September 1936.)

. . . The things I see when I read aren't real, they don't fit the context. If I'm reading a description of some palace, for some reason the main rooms always turn out to be those in the apartment I lived in as a child . . . Take the time I was reading *Trilby*. When I came to the part where I had to find an attic room, without fail it turned out to be one of my neighbor's rooms—in that same house of ours. I noticed it didn't fit the context, but all the same my images led me there automatically. This means I have to spend far more time with a passage if I'm to get some control of things, to reconstruct the images I see. This makes for a tremendous amount of conflict and it becomes difficult for me to read. I'm slowed down, my attention is distracted, and I can't get the important ideas in a passage. Even when I read about circumstances that are entirely new to me, if there happens to be a description, say, of a staircase, it turns out to be one in a house I once lived in. I start to follow it and lose the gist of what I'm reading. What happens is that I just can't read, can't study, for it takes up such an enormous amount of my time . . .

(Record of December 1935.)

Given such a tendency, cognitive functions can hardly proceed normally. The very thought which occasions an image is soon replaced by another— to which the image itself has led; a point is thus reached at which images begin to guide one's thinking, rather than thought itself being the dominant element.

Consider, too, the problem S. had with synonyms, homonyms, and metaphors. We are all familiar with their function in language, the average mind has no problem whatever with them. A person may not even be aware that a thing is variously termed, or if he is aware of it, may feel there is a certain charm in the fact that we can refer to a small child as "child" or "baby"; to a doctor by any of three terms (at least in Russian—*vrach, doktor, medik*); to "commotion" by the synonyms *perepolokh* and *sumatokha;* to a "liar" as either *vrun* or *lgun*. Does anyone find it difficult to grasp the fact that the meaning of a word may change with its context: for example, *ekipazh,* which in Russian means either "cab" or "ship's crew"? Would anyone find it puzzling to read in one passage that the cab (*ekipazh*) stopped at the gates, and then in another passage have the same word turn up in a context such as: "The ship's crew displayed great heroism in the face of a storm with a 10-degree wind force"? Would knowing the expression *spustitsya po lestnitse* ("to go downstairs") make it hard for anyone to grasp that the verb could have a different meaning in another context *spustitsya do bezobraznovo sostoyaniya* ("lapse into unseemly behavior")? Are we at all put off by the fact that *ruchka* can be used to designate not only a child's arm but a door handle, a penholder, and a God knows what else?

The conventional use of language is such that abstraction and generalization are most basic. Hence, people are generally not even aware of problems such as these, or, if they notice them at all, simply pass on without devoting any time to them. Indeed, some linguists believe that language consists just of metaphors and metonyms.* Do these elements hinder our thinking in any way?†

In the case of S.'s figurative, synesthetic thinking, the situation was entirely different. We have already noted the problems he faced if the sound of a word failed to fit its meaning or if the same object were variously termed. Could he possibly agree that a pig in reality had none of the grace he detected in the sound of the word [Russian: *svinya*]; that a biscuit [Russian: *korzhik*] need not be oblong or grooved? Could he even grasp the idea that the words *svinya* and *khavronya,* so different in sound structure, designated the same animal?

S.'s problems with language were even more serious:

. . . Take, for example, the word *ekipazh.*‡ This definitely has to be a cab. So how am I to understand

* Cf. R. Jakobson and M. Halle: *Foundations of Language* (The Hague, Mouton, 1956).

† It is only in unusual circumstances that people have significant difficulty grasping meanings such as these; for example, in the case of deaf and dumb children, to whom the general meaning of words is a major stumbling block. See R. M. Boskis: "Peculiar Features of Speech Development in Children Suffering from a Defect of the Sound Analyzer," *Proceedings of the Academy of Pedagogical Sciences,* RSFSR, XLVIII (1953); and N. G. Morozova: "Training Deaf and Dumb Pupils to Read with Awareness," *Uchpedgiz,* Moscow, 1953.

‡ Word just discussed in a previous paragraph.

right off that it can also mean the crew of a ship? I
have to perform quite an operation in my head, to
block details that come to mind, if I'm to understand
this. What I have to do is to picture to myself not just
a driver or a footman in the cab but an entire staff
manning it. That's the only way I can make sense of it.

. . . And take the expression *to weigh one's words.*
Now how can you weigh words? When I hear the word
*weigh,* I see a large scale—like the one we had in
Rezhitsa in our shop, where they put bread on one
side and a weight on the other. The arrow shifts to one
side, then stops in the middle . . . But what do you
have here—to *weigh one's words!*

. . . Once L. S. Vygotsky's wife said to me: "Can't
you leave Assya for just a minute?"* With that I could
just see her stealing up to the gate and stealthily drop-
ping something there—a child. Now I ask you, can you
really say such a thing?

And then there's the expression to chop wood.† But
*kolot* is something you do with a needle! Yet here's
the word *wood* in the expression. And what about
phrases like *the wind drove the clouds? Drove* to me
suggests a shepherd with a whip; I see his flock and the
dust on the road. I'm confused too by the expression
*the captain's cabin.‡* And when a mother says to her
child, "You've got to do this!" I get confused, for the

* Here the reference is to the verb *podkinut,* which means "to
leave" but may also imply "to abandon." [Tr.]
† In Russian: *kolot drova.* Here *kolot* is a verb, but it can
also be used as a noun, meaning a "prick" or "stab." [Tr.]
‡ *Rubka kapitana:* here meaning "captain's cabin." The noun
*rubka,* however, can also mean "felling" (of wood). [Tr.]

word *sledyet* means to follow someone—I can see it."*
(Record of May 1934.)

This clearly indicates that figurative thinking is not always helpful in understanding language. In S.'s case it was a particular hindrance when he tried to read poetry; in fact, poetry was probably the most difficult thing for him to read.

Many people think that poetry calls for the most graphic kind of thinking. Yet, upon analysis, this idea seems most doubtful, for poetry does not evoke images so much as ideas. The images in a poem merely serve to clothe meaning, the underlying intention of the poem. Hence, to understand a poem, we must be able to grasp the figurative meaning suggested by an image; it is the figurative meaning, not the literal sense of images, that is essential in poetry. What, after all, would we get out of the *Song of Songs* were we to take literally the images used to describe Shulamite—to picture to ourselves the metaphors by which she is described?

S. found that when he tried to read poetry the obstacles to his understanding were overwhelming: each expression gave rise to an image; this, in turn, would conflict with another image that had been evoked. How, then, to break through this chaos

* Though the verb *sledovat* means "to follow," it can also be used in the third person singular to convey necessity or obligation. [Tr.]

of images to the poetry itself. Note, for example, how difficult a poem like the following proved to be.

An old man was standing in a grape trough,
Clutching a pole, stamping grapes with his feet.
But the worker in him, grown fierce with greed,
Eyed that river of wine he so revered.

Sunset came as usual, gigantic it rumbled,
Rocking the grass, the wind pounding the old man's hut.
He stepped out of that low wooden trough,
Barefoot entering his hut, now such a jumble.

N. Tikhonov, *from the Georgian poems*

. . . I saw the old man clearly. He was a little taller than average, had rags wrapped around his legs, and looked something like Leo Tolstoy. He was standing in a place that resembled a garden . . . As for the word *kupel* [here meaning "grape trough"] that's a bunch of grapes. What first appeared was the brown polished barrel of a gun . . . I saw the old man. It seemed as if he were cursing the servant for something. Farther on I saw the river of wine, a dark river since wine [Russian: *vino*] is such a dark word. The river that appeared was one I know in Rezhitsa, near a place called the Mount of Bathsheba . . . Earlier there had been an old ruined castle on this mountain. Behind the mountain I could see some sort of glow—sunrise, apparently. Most likely it was coming up behind the sawmill in Rezhitsa . . . Then I saw some tall grass that began to sway . . . I didn't know what this signified— individual blades of grass, tall grass, sedge . . . I was

standing at the shore and saw all this from a distance
. . . Then the objects grew larger. The figure of the
old man, transparent, rushed past me, swept by like a
zephyr. Through it I could see the grass and to the left,
it seemed, a hut with a tightly fitting roof. The furniture
inside was familiar to me—no doubt the furniture we
had at home. No, I just don't understand this . . .

The impression I got of the poem was rather like
what you'd get if you accidentally overheard a conversation—fragments of images that made no sense
. . . At first it seemed the old man was enraged with the
servant and was kicking him because the servant was
rich, was wearing rope sandals. The servant doesn't
protest, for he loves wine . . . Then the river appeared
to me. After that I gave up trying to follow the poem.
It was a nightmare . . .

(Record of March 1935.)

Three day later the poem was read to him
slowly, stanza by stanza. Then his response was as
follows:

(*First Stanza*): Aha, now I see it differently. He himself is a worker, is greedy, full of awe for that river
of wine flowing from the fruit. Then I heard *in him*.
Does this mean he's a hired laborer? He's undergoing
some terrible experience.

At this point the experimenter explained to him that
the man in the poem is pressing grapes.

Ah, but ever since I was a child I had another image of how that was done. There was a section cut out of a log. My teacher told me this was for *dresten weintzuben.* I took a look through the window of that wooden enclosure and saw how it was all done in this trough. Before I can understand a new image, I have to get rid of an old one that's remained in my mind.

(*Second Stanza*): He walked into that jumble—a mess. But how can this be? There was smoke coming out of the hut. So what's this? As for *rumbled*—I let that pass. It must be because of the raindrops beating down on the grass . . .

He stepped into the hut, and in the room . . . But that's the same room I saw when I was reading Zoshchenko; it comes up in an incident in which, at harvest time, someone proposes to a woman . . . "She sat there and scratched her feet"—and so here's the hut and this is the room . . .

*Sunset rumbled*—that's impossible. A sunset is something idyllic . . . As for *grass rocking,* that's not right. Little blades of grass don't rock; a tree does. And so I saw sedge grass. But if the sunset is idyllic, what's making the grass stir so that it rocks?

The wind pounded the hut! But how can there be any wind during such a sunset? Pounded, pounded—did it shift the hut? Was the hut moved? Ah, it pounded things inside . . . No, that's not possible. But, then, I was still standing outside the hut. It was only when I'd heard the words *Barefoot entering* that the door to the hut opened . . .

I'm very conservative in my use of words. I used to think *prophylactic measures* was an expression that could be used only in medicine, that an *interval* was strictly a musical term. I wondered why people were so quick to use these expressions in other areas. It seemed to me a trick, a sophism . . . No, I'd have to read it through more quickly to get it, so that images won't appear. Otherwise, I see every word . . .

And this is what he made of a few lines from another poem:

[It] Smiled at a bird-cherry tree, sobbed, drenched
The lacquer of cabs, the tremor of trees . . .*

Boris Pasternak

He smiled at a bird-cherry tree. This called up an image of a young man. Then I realized this was taking place on the Metinskaya in Rezhitsa . . . He smiled at it. But right after that there's the word *sobbed*. That is, tears have appeared and are wetting it . . . it means the lines have to do with grief . . . I remembered how some woman went to the crematorium and sat there for hours looking at a portrait . . . That expression *the lacquer of cabs*—it's the lady of the manor driving by in her carriage from the mill at Yuzhatov. I look on. What is she doing? She's looking out of the carriage, trying to see what's wrong there. Why is "he" sad? . . . Then there's the expression *the tremor of trees* [word order

* The verbs are all in the past tense, masculine singular, but they apply to rain; it is the spring rain Pasternak ascribes human emotions to. S. interpreted the content and endings of the verbs as the action of a masculine subject, whereas the subject was masculine in a purely grammatical sense. [Tr.]

reversed in the Russian]. I can see the tremor and then the trees, but when the words are reversed like this, I see a tree and have to make it sway back and forth to understand the phrase itself. This means a lot of work for me.

(Record of March 1938.)

Is it any wonder that this approach, in which each word gave rise to images, kept S. from understanding poetry? S. was fond of dividing poets into two types: simple and complex. And although Pushkin was among those he considered simple, he had marked difficulty following his poetry too. Here we quote verbatim from a letter S. sent us in which he analyzed one of Pushkin's poems.

I confess I found it extremely difficult to be both the experimenter and the subject. But I've tried to be conscientious and disinterested in this. As soon as I read the poem I wrote my commentary and tried to finish it as quickly as possible so that no irrelevant details would slip in.

*To Ogareva, to Whom the Metropolitan Has Sent Fruit from His Garden*

A. PUSHKIN

The metropolitan, that shameless braggart,
Has sent you some of his fruit,
Clearly to convince us he, in truth,
Is God of the gardens.

Small wonder, is it? Kharita
Will conquer decrepitude with a smile;
Driven to a frenzy of desire,
The metropolitan will go wild.

Bewitched by the magic of your glance,
He'll forget about his cross, his duty,
And tenderly begin to chant
Hymns to your heavenly beauty.

I had no problem following the poem. It's simple.
Though I wasn't aware of it, the ideas in the poem
carried me along (which means the style didn't interfere with the way images in the poem developed). In
one of the big rooms in my parents' apartment in
Ravdin's house I saw the beautiful Ogareva sitting in a
tall chair. The left side of her face was clearly illuminated, and behind her I caught sight of our wall clock.
I saw her take the letter out of a basket of fruit she
was holding on her knees. It was at this point I got to
the phrase *to convince us*. I still didn't know who *us*
referred to. *Convince* was clear—but by what means?
Obviously through the letter. At this point a transparent
figure of the God of the gardens, a gray-haired old
man with a flowing beard, emerged from the darkened
corner of the room. I've been trying to find some explanation of how I hit upon this image . . . Now I've
got it! The poem, after all, has to do with the metropolitan. As I read the second stanza I could see who
Pushkin intended with that *us*. It was the young Pushkin and two of his friends who were standing on the
street near the window of the house laughing and
joking maliciously. Pushkin was coming out with a

stream of witticisms as he stood there pointing to the window. I didn't have time to listen in on what he was saying since I had already gotten to the third stanza.

Here that image of the decrepit *God of the gardens* became "more compact" (before this his figure had been transparent). I saw him dressed in a black surplice; he was standing gazing at Ogareva and seemed to be imploring her, while she sat there, her hand holding the letter dropped in a gesture of helplessness. The large gold cross on his breast slowly began to fade as he lifted his head and looked at her with lusterless eyes that seemed to have some glimmer to them. (Aha! Now his whole figure has become clear!) In his hoarse bass voice he began to sing a romance in the style of a church hymn. Ogareva looked at him with an expression that was both astonished and confused.

Then the ceiling of the room, which had been covered with some sort of glossy paper, was transformed into a milky-white cloud. Against this I could see the beautiful face of a woman with loose, fair hair, a face familiar to me from childhood, when I first began studying at the Hebrew school. Then she seemed to me to be "the voice of God" speaking through the prophets. In Hebrew she is called *Bas-keil*—the daughter of the voice (of God) . . .

(From S.'s letter of November 1937.)

This, then, is what a "simple" poem gave rise to for S. Although the images that appeared to him did not prevent him from following the poem, they could hardly be said to have helped him.

Thus far, we have been dealing with S.'s responses to imagery, narrative prose, and poetry. How did he interpret explanatory material and abstract, scientific literature? What effect did his figurative, synesthetic thinking have on his grasp of this type of material?

Let us turn now from the poetry of Tikhonov and Pasternak to examples of scientific writing which S. tried to understand. We will begin with a simple sentence S. was asked to interpret. The sentence read: "The work got under way normally." Could there be anything complicated about such a sentence? We would have thought S. could have no trouble with it, but he found it very difficult to grasp.

. . . I read that "the work got under way normally." As for *work,* I see that work is going on . . . there's a factory . . . But there's that word *normally.* What I see is a big, ruddy-cheeked woman, a *normal* woman . . . Then the expression *get under way.* Who? What is all this? You have industry . . . that is, a factory, and this normal woman—but how does all this fit together? How much I have to get rid of just to get the simple idea of the thing!

(Record of December 1935.)

His problem is familiar to us by now: each word he read produced images that distracted him and blocked the meaning of a sentence. When it came to texts that contained descriptions of complex relationships, formulations of rules, or explanations of causal connections, S. fared even worse.

For example, I read him a simple rule such as the following, which any schoolboy could easily understand: "If carbon dioxide is present above a vessel, the greater its pressure, the faster it dissolves in water." Consider the obstacles this abstract, yet nonetheless uncomplicated, statement presented.

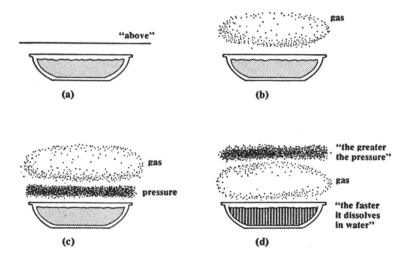

When you gave me this sentence I immediately saw the vessel. As for that *above* that is mentioned, it's here . . . I see a line (a). Above the vessel a small cloud

that's moving in an upward direction. That's the gas (b).
I read further: "the greater the pressure"—so the gas
rises . . . Then there's something dense here—the pressure (c). But the pressure is greater—it rises higher
. . . As for the phrase "the faster it dissolves in water"
—the water has become heavy (d) . . . And the gas—
you say "the higher the pressure"—it's moved steadily
higher . . . So what does it all mean? If the pressure
is higher, how can it dissolve in water?

(Record of December 1935.)

Seemingly, S. had none too easy a time of it
understanding the simple idea contained in this
law. Details which other people would overlook,
or which would remain on the periphery of awareness, took on independent value in his mind, giving
rise to images that tended to scatter meaning.

Up to now we have been dealing with more or
less concrete material: descriptions of objects and
events which could conceivably be visualized mentally—at least in part. What was S.'s reaction to
abstract ideas which he could not visualize—defini-
tions of complex relationships, abstract concepts
that have been worked out over the course of cen-
turies? These ideas exist; we learn them in school;
yet we cannot visualize their content. S., however,
had told us many times: "I can only understand
what I can visualize."

Abstract ideas meant another round of problems and torments for him, another series of attempts to reconcile the incompatible. Note how he struggled to grasp these ideas.

. . . *Infinity*—that means what has always been. But what came before this? What is to follow? No, it's impossible to see this . . .

In order for me to grasp the meaning of a thing, I have to see it . . . Take the word *nothing*. I read it and thought it must be very profound. I thought it would be better to call *nothing* something . . . for I see this *nothing* and it is something . . . If I'm to understand any meaning that is fairly deep, I have to get an image of it right away. So I turned to my wife and asked her what *nothing* meant. But it was so clear to her that she simply said: "*Nothing* means there is nothing." I understood it differently. I saw this *nothing* and felt she must be wrong. The logic we use, for example. It's been worked out on the basis of years of experience. I can see how it has developed, and what it means to me is that one has to rely on his own sensations of things. If *nothing* can appear to a person, that means it is something. That's where the trouble comes in . . .

When I hear it said, for example, that water is colorless, I remember how my father once had to cut down a tree at the edge of the Bezymyannaya Stream because it blocked the flow of the current . . . I began to think and wonder what *Bezymyannaya Stream* could mean

[Russian: *bezymyannaya,* "nameless"]. It means the stream has no name . . .

What pointless images come up on account of a single word. Take the word *something,* for example. For me this is a dense cloud of steam that has the color of smoke. When I hear the word *nothing,* I also see a cloud, but one that is thinner, completely transparent. And when I try to seize a particle of this *nothing,* I get the most minute particles of *nothing.*

(Record of December 1935.)

How odd and yet how familiar these experiences are. They are inevitable for any adolescent who, having grown used to thinking in terms of graphic images, suddenly finds there is a world of abstract ideas to be mastered. He is bound to be confused by the questions these pose: What do we mean by *nothing* when something always exists? What does *eternity* mean? What came before? What will follow? Similarly with *infinity*—what will there be after infinity? These concepts exist and are taught to us in school. Yet how can we picture them in our minds? And if it is impossible to imagine them, what do they mean?

These are the questions that perplex and overwhelm young people when they realize that abstract ideas cannot be understood in graphic terms; they are thus forced to grapple with ideas that seem so contradictory. This soon ceases to be a problem for the adolescent, however, for he shifts from thinking in concrete terms to dealing with abstractions; the role graphic images once played in his thinking is replaced by certain accepted ideas about the meaning of words. His thinking becomes verbal and logical in nature, and graphic images remain on the periphery of consciousness, since they are of no help in understanding abstract concepts.

Once we have made the transition to another level of thought, the problem of abstractions is just a memory of a painful experience we had in the past. S., though, could not make the transition as rapidly as others. He was unable to grasp an idea unless he could actually see it, and so he tried to visualize the idea of "nothing," to find an image with which to depict "infinity." And he persisted in these agonizing attempts all his life, forever coping with a basically adolescent conflict that made it impossible for him to cross that "accursed" threshold to a higher level of thought.

The images abstract concepts such as the above evoked were of no help to him. What could he really deduce from the fact that upon hearing the word *eternity,* an image of some ancient figure, of God no doubt, whom he had learned of from Bible stories, would appear to him? At times, instead of images he would see "puffs of steam," "splashes," and "lines." What did they represent? The content of the abstract ideas S. was trying to visualize? What did he derive from the images which, as we know, he would see in response to the sounds of a word he was not familiar with? It is difficult to say whether these images were of any help to him in understanding an idea. But they continued to emerge, crowding together and taking up much of his conscious awareness.

When I read newspapers, some things are clear to me. I have a good understanding of everything that has to do with economic affairs. But there are other ideas I can't grasp right away, ones I only get much later. Why? The answer is clear: I just can't visualize them. If I can't see it, it just doesn't penetrate . . . Even when I listen to works of music, I feel the taste of them on my tongue; if I can't, I don't understand the music. This means I have to experience not only abstract ideas, but even music, through a physical sense of taste . . . If it's simply a matter of learning a phone number, though I repeat it, I won't really know the number unless I've tasted it. Otherwise I have to listen to it again, to let it penetrate. So where do I stand with regard to abstract ideas? When I hear the word *pain,* for example, I see bands—little round objects, and fog. It's the fog that has to do with the abstractness of the word . . .

(Record of December 1935.)

S. tried to convert everything into images; when this proved impossible, into "puffs of steam" or "lines." And all his effort was expended in trying to arrive at meaning through these visual forms. There was also another obstacle in that the longer he thought about a thing, the more persistently would those old, tenacious images of early childhood come to mind: images of Rezhitsa, of his home, where as a very young child he had been read stories from the Bible, and where for the first time he tried to make sense out of ideas that were so difficult for his mind to grasp. Consider, for example, his confusion with the following passage:

With respect to art, we know that it flourished in periods when there was no corresponding growth in the development of society as a whole and therefore in the material base of the latter, which, as it were, constituted the framework of its organization.

S. proceeded to interpret it in this way:

It started off well enough . . . For some reason I had an image of antiquity—ruins of places where Aristotle and Socrates once lived. But what I really saw was Chaim Petukh's home, where I had once studied about antiquity. When I looked at pictures of ruins there, I'd see the Temple of the Maccabees. Yet it was art we were talking about. I always get an image of Nero when I think about those times; also Caligula's senate meeting in our synagogue. For, after all, it's the sort of place in which the Sanhedrin met . . . I just can't make anything out of this whole sentence . . . Then "public life"—that is, the "social mentality"—was not reflected in art . . . The social and class relationships within society were not reflected in the art of the time. As for *framework,** that must mean the carcass of something.

Now, as I read it over a second time, it's clear! Even the word *framework* seems secondary. Still, the phrase about "the material base of society" is abstract to me. It's a cloud.

(Record of June 1936.)

On the whole, however, S. did learn to master most of what he had to in life: he associated with people, attended courses, took examinations. However, each attempt to move beyond the unsteady plateaus of his level of understanding to some higher awareness proved arduous, for at each step he had to contend with superfluous images and sensations. There is no question that S.'s figurative, synesthetic thinking had both its high and its low points, and that both were bound up with distinct strengths and limitations.

* The word in Russian is literally "skeleton"; hence his confusion. [Tr.]

# 6

## *His Control of Behavior*

We have devoted a number of pages to describing the strong and weak points of S.'s intelligence. Let us consider the influence of the strengths and weaknesses of his imagination on his control of his own behavior.

### THE OBJECTIVE DATA

Probably all of us can recall some simple test we made when we were children to try to prove the power of our imagination. For example, the sort of test a child might make who stands with his hand outstretched, his fingers gripping a string to which a little weight is attached. The child imagines that his hand, which is actually still, has begun to move in a circular motion. Slowly the weight does in fact begin to move until it picks up speed and whirls around in a distinctly circular motion. What happens is that the object is set in motion by the force of the child's imagination. Psychologists, aware of the mechanisms behind the "ideo-motor" act, believe that most of what is involved in that mysterious act known as "thought reading" can be explained as a reading of the expressions imagination has aroused on the face of the person being observed. How much evidence, too, there is in the current field of psychosomatic medicine to indicate that in the Middle Ages a powerful imagination was sufficient to produce stigmata in a hysterical woman; that, in general, imagination can induce changes in somatic processes. And the descriptions of experiences the Indian yogi have attained indicate how much remains to be explored with respect to the force of imagination.

Is it any wonder, then, that with his exceptionally vivid imagination S. would inevitably prove capable of inducing in himself certain bodily movements, that by virtue of power of his imagination he would have far greater control over his own body processes than the ordinary man? He put it all quite simply:

If I want something to happen, I simply picture it in my mind. I don't have to exert any effort to accomplish it—it just happens.

(Record of May 1934.)

Nonetheless, could an experimenter simply take him at his word and not attempt to verify the limits and the possibilities of control he had over his body? Tests indicated this was not idle talk on S.'s part; he could arbitrarily regulate his heart activity and his body temperature. And he had a considerable range of control over these.

The following is the demonstration he gave us of how he could alter his pulse rate. At rest, his pulse was normally 70–72. But after a slight pause he could make it accelerate until it had increased to 80–96, and finally to 100. We also saw him reverse the rate. His pulse began to slow down, and after it had dropped to its previous rate continued to decrease until it was a steady 64–66. When we asked him how he did this, he replied:

What do you find so strange about it? I simply see myself running after a train that has just begun to pull out. I have to catch up with the last car if I'm to make it. Is it any wonder then my heartbeat increases? After that, I saw myself lying in bed, perfectly still, trying to fall asleep . . . I could see myself begin to drop off . . . my breathing became regular, my heart started to beat more slowly and evenly . . .

And here is another experiment he performed for us:

Would you like to see me raise the temperature of my right hand and lower that of my left? Let's begin . . .
(Record of June 1938.)

We used a skin thermometer to check the temperature of both hands and found they were the same. After a minute had passed, then another, he said: "All right, begin!" We attached the thermometer to the skin on his right hand and found that the temperature had risen two degrees. As for his left hand, after S. paused for a minute and then announced he was ready, the reading showed that the temperature of his left hand had dropped one and a half degrees.

What could this mean? How was it possible for him to control the temperature of his body at will?

No, there's nothing to be amazed at. I saw myself put my right hand on a hot stove . . . Oi, was it hot! So, naturally, the temperature of my hand increased. But I was holding a piece of ice in my left hand. I could see it there and began to squeeze it. And, of course, my hand got colder . . .

(Record of June 1938.)

Could he also use this as a means of overcoming pain? S. had told us about the methods he used to avoid experiencing severe pain:

Let's say I'm going to the dentist. You know how pleasant it is to sit there and let him drill your teeth. I used to be afraid to go. But now it's all so simple. I sit there and when the pain starts I feel it . . . it's a tiny, orange-red thread . . . I'm upset because I know that if this keeps up, the thread will widen until it turns into a dense mass . . . So I cut the thread, make it smaller and smaller, until it's just a tiny point. And the pain disappears.

Later I tried a different method. I'd sit in the chair but imagine it wasn't really me but someone else. I, S., would merely stand by and observe "him" getting his teeth drilled. Let him feel the pain . . . It doesn't hurt me, you understand, but "him." I just don't feel any pain.

(Record of January 1935.)

Admittedly, this was never verified under controlled conditions. However, we did ascertain, in the presence of some of our colleagues, that S.

could alter the processes whereby he adapted to the dark by visualizing himself in a room that had different degrees of illumination. And when he imagined he was hearing a piercing sound, he evidenced a cochlear-pupil reflex. Further, his electro-encephalogram showed a distinct depression of the alpha waves when he imagined that a blazing light from a 500-watt bulb was flashing in his eyes.*

Physiological research which was conducted at the Physiology Laboratory of the Neurology Clinic, All-Union Institute of Experimental Medicine, by S. A. Kharitonov and his associates yielded few indications of the possible mechanisms behind these phenomena. No appreciable changes were found in S.'s threshold of touch; however, he did experience touch in terms of graphic (synesthetic) images. His thresholds of sensitivity to taste and to smell decreased, and those of visual adaptation were markedly changed: he required more time to adapt to the dark. Stimulation of the skin with Frey's filaments produced no significant change in threshold, but instead of a pointed sensation of touch, S. experienced waves that began to extend until they had encompassed large areas of his skin. His skin sensitivity indicated heightened inertia, whereas certain

* These experiments were carried out with the collaboration of S. A. Kharitonov, N. V. Rayeva, S. D. Rolle, and A. I. Rudnik. We gratefully acknowledge their assistance.

features peculiar to his experience of touch point to a prevalence of protopathic sensitivity. The thresholds of his optical chronaxie were within the range of normal, but the subjective sensations aroused in response to electrical stimulation of the skin were exceptionally severe (particularly when one considers that an increase in the intensity of stimuli usually does not produce a corresponding increase in sensation). Once the threshold changes, it remains at the same level for a considerable period, individual peculiarities of response being less apparent in the threshold values than in the dynamics of the excitation that has been caused.

Naturally, we would have put great store by what objective research on S.'s vegetative, sensory, and electrophysiological reactions would reveal. Such research, however, contributed negligible and rather indirect information and did not bring us a much closer understanding of the remarkable phenomena described in this account of S. However, it sometimes happens that objective analysis of the facts one is investigating does not add up to one's expectations.

Let us return, now, to our account and consider the psychology of the phenomena we have been concerned with, supplementing what we already know with information on some curious traits that were observed in S.

## A FEW WORDS ABOUT MAGIC

We have been dealing thus far with the facts as we saw them as objective observers. But what was S.'s perspective on them? In order to make his viewpoint clear, we will have to digress somewhat and consider some points that were not touched on earlier in this account.

With each individual there is a dividing line between imagination and reality; for most of us whose imaginations have distinct limits, this is fairly clear-cut. In S.'s case the borderline between the two had broken down, for the images his imagination conjured up took on the feel of reality.

This is the way things tended to work when I was a boy and going to Hebrew school. I'd wake up and see that it was morning and that I had to get up . . . I'd look at the clock and think: "No, there's still time, I can stay in bed for a while." And I'd continue to see the hands of the clock pointing at 7:30, which meant it was still early. Suddenly my mother would come in and say: "What, you haven't left yet? Why, it'll soon be nine." Well, how was I to know that? I saw the big hand pointing down—according to the clock, it was 7:30.

(Record of October 1934.)

The boy's vivid imagination broke down the boundary between the real and the imaginary; and this lack of distinction between the two produced quite unusual behavior on his part.

And if the line between imagination and reality breaks down, isn't it possible that the distinction between one's image of oneself and that of another might be effaced, or at least weakened?

In S.'s case, this tendency was in evidence as far back as early childhood. We are aware of course that "magical" thinking is natural to young children, that it is a simple matter for them to perform some trick of the imagination, say, whereby they keep their teacher from calling on them. All it takes is for the child to grip his desk firmly and think to himself that his teacher's glance has already passed him. It doesn't always work, but the child may think: "All the same, maybe it will help." Naturally, S. went through this in the early grades. But whereas such thinking is generally a passing phase and remains merely as a memory of chidlhood, as an experience somewhere between childish play and a pleasant naïve sort of "magic," with S. the tendency persisted. And he himself couldn't really say whether he believed in it or not.

We had a teacher named Friedrich Adamovich and we used to play tricks on him. "Who did it?" he'd ask. He'd walk into the room, and I'd think: "Now he'll catch me." With all my might I'd fix him with a look and he'd think: "No, he hasn't done anything . . ."

I'd see him turn away from me and look elsewhere. "No, he won't get me for this," I'd think.

Many times he caught himself in acts which seemed to be a play of imagination but which he, nonetheless, tended to take quite seriously. As he put it:

To me there's no great difference between the things I imagine and what exists in reality. Often, if I imagine something is going to happen, it does. Take the time I began arguing with a friend that the cashier in the store was sure to give me too much change. I imagined it to myself in detail, and she actually did give me too much—change of 20 rubles instead of 10 . . . Of course I realize it's just chance, coincidence, but deep down I also think it's because I saw it that way . . . And if I don't manage to make a thing happen, it seems to me it's either because I got tired, or distracted, or because the other person's will was fixed on something else.

(Record of January 1938.)

Sometimes I even think I can cure myself if I imagine it clearly enough. I can even treat other people. I know that when I start to get sick, I imagine the illness is passing . . . there, it's gone, I'm well. And I don't actually get sick.

One time when I was planning to go to Samara, Misha [his son] developed stomach pains. We called in a doctor, but he couldn't figure out what was wrong with him . . . Yet it was so simple. I had given him something that was cooked with lard. I could see the pieces of lard in his stomach . . . I thought to myself I'd help him. I wanted him to digest them . . . I pictured it in my mind and saw the lard dissolving in his stomach. And Misha got better. Of course, I know this isn't the way it happened . . . yet I did see it all.

(Record of February 1938.)

How many moments there were in his life of naïve "magical" thinking when his imagination succeeded in convincing him of something, even though his reason thrust it aside. Some grain of doubt would remain; in some remote part of his awareness he continued to feel: perhaps it really is true? How many odd nooks and crannies there were to the man's mind where imagination would become reality for him.

# 7

## *His Personality*

Let us now turn to the last section of our account, which, though it is the one we know least about, is probably the most interesting.

An entire body of writings, though not of any considerable scope, is to be found on outstanding mnemonists. Thus, psychologists are familiar with the names Inodi and Diamandi, and the literature on the Japanese mnemonist Ishihara. However, the psychologists who wrote about these mnemonists dealt only with their memory and imagination, their amazing ability to do mental calculations; none provided any information on these people's personalities.

What sort of man was Inodi? How did Diamandi's personal life develop? What distinct personality features did Ishihara exhibit? What was his manner of life?

The basic concepts of classical psychology made for a sharp disjunction between theories about specific psychic functions and theories of personality structure, the implication being, apparently, that individual personality features are hardly dependent on the nature of these psychic functions; that an individual who demonstrates striking peculiarities of memory in the laboratory may in everyday life be no different than anyone else.

Yet is this true? Is it reasonable to think that the existence of an extraordinarily developed figurative memory, of synesthesia, has no effect on an individual's personality structure? Can a person who "sees" everything; who cannot understand a thing unless an impression of it "leaks" through all his sense organs; who must feel a telephone number on the tip of his tongue before he can remember it —can he possibly develop as others do? Could it be said of him that his experiences in attending school, making friends, taking up a career in life were pretty much those of other people; that his inner world, his life history developed quite like those of others? From the outset, such an assumption seems highly unlikely to us.

An individual whose conscious awareness is such that a sound becomes fused with a sense of color and taste; for whom each fleeting impression engenders a vivid, inextinguishable image; for whom words have quite different meanings than they do for us—such a person cannot mature in the same way others do, nor will his inner world, his life history tend to be like others'. A person who has "seen" and experienced life synesthetically cannot have the same grasp of things the rest of us have, nor is he likely to experience himself or other people as we might.

Precisely how did S.'s personality and life history develop? Let us begin the history of his development with an incident from his early childhood:

It's morning . . . I have to go to school. Soon it'll be eight o'clock. I have to get up, get dressed, put on my coat and hat, my galoshes . . . I can't stay in bed. I start to get angry, for I see I have to go to school . . . But why shouldn't "he" go? No, I won't go. He'll get up and get dressed. There he is, he's getting his coat and cap, putting on his galoshes. Now he's gone. So everything's as it should be. I stay home, and "he" goes off. But suddenly my father walks in and says: "It's so late, and you haven't left for school yet?"

(Record of October 1934.)

The boy was a dreamer whose fantasies were embodied in images that were all too vivid, constituting in themselves another world, one through which he transformed the experiences of everyday life. He thus tended to lose sight of the distinction between what formed part of reality and what he himself could "see."

This was a habit I had for quite some time; perhaps even now I still do it. I'd look at a clock and for a long while continue to see the hands fixed just as they were, and not realize time had passed . . . That's why I'm often late.

(Record of October 1934.)

How, after all, was S. to adjust to rapidly shifting impressions when the images that emerged from these were so vivid they could easily become reality for him?

They always called me a *kalter nefesh* [Yiddish: "a cold duck"]. Say there's a fire and I haven't yet begun to understand what a fire is (for I would have had to have seen it first, you know). If at that moment I still had not seen a fire, I'd react cold-bloodedly to the news.

(Record of June 1934.)

We know that a creative imagination—the kind of imagination that makes for great inventors— operates in a manner that is closely in touch with reality. But there is another type of imagination whose activity is not directed toward the external world, but is nourished by desire and becomes a substitute for action by making action seem pointless. Indeed, how many idle dreamers are there who live in a world of imagination, transforming their lives into a "waking dream," their time given up to daydreaming.

Given S.'s diffuse synesthetic experiences and exquisitely sensitive images, how could he not become a dreamer? His were not the sort of dreams that just led to idleness; they became a substitute for action in that they were based on his experiences of himself which were converted into images. This is a quality of fantasy we noted in the incident referred to several paragraphs earlier.

I had to go to school . . . I saw myself here, while "he" was to go off to school. I'm angry with "him"—why is he taking so long to get ready?

And this is another incident he recalled from childhood:

I'm eight years old. We're moving to a new apartment. I don't want to go. My brother takes me by the hand and leads me to the cab waiting outside. I see the driver there munching a carrot. But I don't want to go . . . I stay behind in the house—that is, I see how "he" stands at the window of my old room. He's not going anywhere.

(Record of October 1934.)

This kind of split between the "I" who issues orders and the "he" who carries them out (whom the "I" in S. visualized) persisted throughout his life. "He" would go off when it was necessary; "he" would recall things; the "I" would merely instruct, direct, control. If we had not been aware of the psychological mechanisms behind those vivid graphic "visions" of S.'s which we have examined in such detail here, we might easily have been led to take him for one of those "split personalities" psychiatrists deal with, and with whom S.'s particular kind of "cutting himself off" had so little in common.

His ability to "see" himself in this way, to "cut himself off," to convert his experiences and activity into an image of another person who carried out his instructions—all this was of enormous help to him in regulating his own behavior. We had a glimpse of this earlier when we observed how he was able to control his vegetative processes and eliminate pain by transferring it to another person.

Yet sometimes his "cutting himself off" in this way interfered with his having complete control of his behavior. The following situation is indicative.

Take the situation here. I'm sitting in your apartment preoccupied with my own thoughts. You, being a good host, ask: "How do you like these cigarettes?" "So-so, fair . . ." That is, I'd never say that, but "he" might. It's not tactful, but I can't explain the slip to him. For "I" understand things, but "he" doesn't. If I'm distracted, "he" says things he oughtn't to.

(Record of October 1934.)

In circumstances such as these, a slight distraction was all it took for the "he" S. saw to slip out of control and begin to operate automatically. There were many instances too in which images that came to the surface in S.'s mind steered him away from the subject of a conversation. At such moments his remarks would be cluttered with details and irrelevancies; he would become verbose, digress endlessly, and finally have to strain to get back to the subject of the conversation.

S. knew he was verbose; he knew he had to be on the alert to keep to a topic. At times, though, this was scarcely possible. I, as his observer, and the stenographers who transcribed our conversations were acutely aware of this; in putting this account together I realized how difficult it was to single out what was essential in my conversations with S. from his endless digressions. He explained his tendency to digress in this way:

All this makes it impossible for me to stick to the subject we're discussing. It's not that I'm talkative. Say you ask me about a horse. There's also its color and taste I have to consider. And this produces such a mass of impressions that if "I" don't get the situation in hand, we won't get anywhere with the discussion. "He," you see, has no sense of having gotten off the track. I have to deal not only with the word *horse* but with its taste, the yard it's penned in—which I can't seem to get away from myself . . . It was only recently that I learned to follow a conversation and stick to the subject.

(Record of May 1939.)

How many instances there were also in which the vivid images he saw conflicted with reality, preventing him from carrying out an action he was otherwise well prepared for.

I had to go to court on some business . . . a very simple case which I ought to have won. I prepared what I was going to say . . . I could see the whole court scene. (I can't deal with things any other way.) . . . There was the large courtroom: the rows of chairs, the judge's table on the right. I stood at the left and spoke. Everyone was satisfied with the evidence I had given and I won . . . But in fact it proved to be entirely different from what I had expected. When I entered the courtroom, the judge wasn't sitting on the right but on the left, so that I had to speak from the other side of the room . . . It wasn't at all like what I had seen, and I just lost my head. I couldn't put my points across, and, naturally, I lost the case.

(Record of May 1939.)

How often it happened that S.'s striking images failed to coincide with reality; how often, having come to rely on them, he would find he was helpless to deal with circumstances. The incident in court was a particularly vivid example, but it was typical of the kinds of incidents S. encountered all through life. It was precisely his helplessness at these times which, as he so often complained, led people to take him for a dull, awkward, somewhat absent-minded fellow.

However, his unstable grasp of reality, and the realistic overtones of his fantasies, had a far more profound effect on his personality development. For he lived in wait of something that he assumed was to come his way, and gave himself up to dreaming and "seeing" far more than to functioning in life. The sense he had that something particularly fine was about to happen remained with him throughout his life—something which would solve all his problems and make his life simple and clear. He "saw" this and waited . . . Thus, everything he did in life was merely "temporary," what he had to do until the expected would finally come to pass.

I read a great deal and always identified myself with one of the heroes. For I saw them, you know. Even at eighteen I couldn't understand how one friend of mine was content to train to become an accountant, another a commercial traveler. For what's important in life isn't a profession but something fine, something grand that is to happen to me . . . If at eighteen or twenty I'd thought I was ready to marry and a countess or princess had agreed to marry me—even that wouldn't have impressed me. Perhaps I was destined for something greater? . . . Whatever I did, whether writing articles, becoming a film star—it was just a temporary thing.

At one point I studied the stock market, and when I showed that I had a good memory for prices on the exchange, I became a broker. But it was just something I did for a while to make a living. As for real life— that's something else again. But it all took place in dreams, not in reality . . .

I was passive for the most part, didn't understand that time was moving on. All the jobs I had were simply work I was doing "in the meantime." The feeling I had was: "I'm only twenty-five, only thirty—I've got my whole life ahead of me." In 1917 I was content to go off to the provinces. I decided to get in with the movement. So I was in the Proletcult, ran a printing shop, became a reporter, lived a special sort of life for a time. But even now I realize time's passing and that I might have accomplished a great deal—but I don't work. That's the way I've always been.

(Record of December 1937.)

Thus, he continued to be disorganized, changing jobs dozens of time—all of them merely "temporary." At his father's bidding he entered music school; later he became a vaudeville actor; then an efficiency expert; and then a mnemonist. At some point, recalling that he knew Hebrew and Aramaic, he took advantage of ancient sources in these languages and began to treat people with herbs.

He had a family—a fine wife and a son who was a success—but this, too, he perceived as though through a haze. Indeed, one would be hard put to say which was more real for him: the world of imagination in which he lived, or the world of reality in which he was but a temporary guest.

Psychology has yet to become a science that is capable of dealing with the really vital aspects of human personality. It has yet to learn to depict the nature of personality in such a way that the function of each individual trait could be seen in its relation to the total personality structure. Similarly, it has yet to reach a point at which the laws of personality development would be as precise and intelligible as those which apply to the synthesis of complex chemical substances.

The development of such a psychology is a job for the future, and at present it is difficult to say how many decades it will be before we achieve it. For the progress that must be made if we are to have a scientific psychology of personality entails numerous turns off the main line of study, many areas of inquiry that will prove difficult to approach. But there is no doubt that research into the way an imbalance of individual aspects of development affects the formation of personality structure, a description of the process through which a personality "syndrome" is created, will constitute one important method in the approaches used.

Perhaps this account of a man who "saw" everything will play some part in the difficult course that lies ahead.